ANESTHESIA AND THE CARDIOVASCULAR SYSTEM

W0105738

DEVELOPMENTS IN CRITICAL CARE MEDICINE AND ANESTHESIOLOGY

ANESTHESIA AND THE CARDIOVASCULAR SYSTEM

Annual Utah postgraduate course in anesthesiology 1984

edited by

THEODORE H. STANLEY, MD and W. CLAYTON PETTY, MD
Department of Anesthesiology
The University of Utah Medical School
Salt Lake City, Utah, USA

Distributors

for the United States and Canada: Kluwer Boston, Inc., 190 Old Derby Street, Hingham, MA 02043, USA
for all other countries: Kluwer Academic Publishers Group, Distribution Center, P.O.Box 322, 3300 AH Dordrecht, The Netherlands

Library of Congress Cataloging in Publication Data

Main entry under title:
Anesthesia and the cardiovascular system.

  (Developments in critical care medicine and
anaesthesiology)
  1. Anesthesia—Complications and sequelae—
Congresses. 2. Cardiovascular system—Diseases—
Complications and sequelae—Congresses. I. Stanley,
Theodore H. II. Petty, W. Clayton. III. Series.
RD87.3.C37A54   1984   617'.96   83-24928

ISBN-13: 978-94-010-9001-8   e-ISBN-13: 978-94-009-5668-1
DOI: 10.1007/978-94-009-5668-1

Copyright

Table of contents

VI

Contributors

Estafanous, F.G., MD, Department of Cardiothoracic Anesthesia, Cleveland Clinic Foundation, Cleveland OH 44106, USA

Glass, D.D., MD, Department of Anesthesiology, Dartmouth Hitchcock Medical Center, Hanover, NH 03755, USA

Hackel, A., MD, Department of Anesthesia, Stanford University Medical Center, Stanford, CA 94305, USA

Katz, R.L., MD, Department of Anesthesiology, UCLA School of Medicine, Los Angeles, CA 90024, USA

Lange, de, S., M.B.B.S, FFARCS, PhD, Department of Anesthesiology, Academisch Ziekenhuis Leiden, Rijnsburgerweg 10, 2333 AA Leiden, The Netherlands

Longnecker, D.E., MD, Department of Anesthesiology, University of Virginia Medical Center, Charlottesville, VA 22908

Mangano, D.T., PhD, MD, Veterans Administration Medical Center, Department of Anesthesiology at UCSF, San Francisco, CA 92161, USA

Pace, N.L., MD, Department of Anesthesiology, University of Utah College, Salt Lake City, UT 84132, USA

Petty, W.C., MD, Department of Anesthesiology, The University of Utah, Medical School, Salt Lake City, UT 84132, USA

Reves, J.G., MD, Department of Anesthesiology, University of Alabama School of Medicine, Birmingham, AL 35294, USA

Rosenthal, M.H., MD, Department of Anesthesia, Stanford University Medical School, Stanford, CA 943005, USA

Tinker, J.H., MD, Department of Anesthesia, University of Iowa Hospitals and Clinics, Iowa City, IA 52240, USA

Wong, K.C., MD, PhD, University of Utah School of Medicine, Department of Anesthesiology, Salt Lake City, UT 84132, USA

ANESTHESIA AND THE CARDIOVASCULAR SYSTEM

PREOPERATIVE EVALUATION OF THE PATIENT WITH CARDIAC DISEASE
PERIOPERATIVE ALTERATION OF LEFT VENTRICULAR FUNCTION

DENNIS T. MANGANO, M.D., Ph.D

Coronary artery disease (CAD) continues to be a significant problem
in the United States as substantiated by the following statistics.

10,000,000	patients with CAD
4,000,000	patients with previous MIs
1,300,000	new MIs/year
700,000	deaths(CAD)/year
400,000	cardiac catheterizations/year
150,000	CABG surgeries/year

It appears that the prognosis (medical or surgical) in CAD is
related to the development and severity of:

1. dysrhythmias
2. myocardial infarction
3. ventricular dysfunction

Preoperative assessment of the significance of these is a critical part
of our management.

THE SIGNIFICANCE OF DYSRHYTHMIAS IN CAD

1. Incidence. With acute myocardial infarction virtually all
patients develop premature ventricular contractions within the first
five days. Within 1-3 weeks following infarction, 73-94% of patients
develop one or more dysrhythmias. With chronic CAD, the incidence of
patients in whom dysrhythmia is the predominant manifestation is
unknown. It is known, however, that the most common dysrhythmias with
chronic CAD are premature ventricular contractions (PVCs). Also, if
chronic PVCs are frequent, multiform, or R-on-T, they are predictive of
multivessel disease or significant ventricular dysfunction.

2. _Detection_. Detection of dysrhythmias depends on the duration of observation and the degree of stress.

Test	Incidence of Ventricular Dysrhythmias
EKG-rest (<1 minute)	14%
EKG-rest (1 hour observation)	50%
EKG-routine activity (24 hour observation)	88%
EKG-stress testing (<1 hour)	52-61%

Although 24 hour monitoring detects ventricular tachycardia approximately twice as often as stress testing, in 10% of the patients, serious dysrhythmias (VT, VF) are detected only with stress testing.

3. _Prognosis_. The most serious dysrhythmias are ventricular fibrillation and tachycardia, and complex PVCs (R-on-T, multiform, repetitive). These carry the greatest risk of sudden death and are predictive of multivessel disease. Also significant are the conduction disturbances: complete heart block, Mobitz II and bundle branch block (mortality 10 to 70%). Acute atrial dysrhythmias are usually indicative of concurrent disease, and are associated with significant risk if accompanied by acute ischemia or left ventricular failure.

4. _Perioperative Risk_. In patients with and without CAD, perioperative dysrhythmias commonly occur (17.9 to 61.7%), and are usually associated with stimulation, CO_2 elevation, hypertension, potassium loss, digitalis therapy and specific anesthetics. Most of these dysrhythmias are supraventricular or PVCs, and few (<1%) are associated with serious sequelae.

In patients with heart disease (CAD, hypertensive, valvular and congenital) or pre-existing dysrhythmias, the incidence of perioperative dysrhythmias (benign and serious) is increased by as much as 3-fold. The type of heart disease (CAD vs valvular) and the severity of the disease (NYHA II vs IV) appear to be the most critical factors. More informative data are lacking.

It thus seems reasonable to conclude that those patients with CAD who are at highest risk of developing serious perioperative dysrhythmias have: (1) prior infarction complicated by serious dysrhythmias, or (2) evidence of ventricular dysfunction, or (3) recurrent or persistent dysrhythmias detected with the rest or exercise EKG.

THE SIGNIFICANCE OF INFARCTION IN CAD

1. <u>Incidence</u>. Approximately 4 million people in the United States have had one or more myocardial infarctions. Each year, 1.3 million patients develop a new myocardial infarction.

2. <u>Detection</u>. The hallmarks of the clinical diagnosis are history, EKG and serum enzymes. The classical findings are well known and will not be discussed. But of note are the following:

    a. History - most patients have angina with infarction. However, 20-33% of infarcts are painless, and 35-90% have no prodromal symptoms. Silent extension of MIs has been reported in up to 57% of patients.

    b. EKG - with infarction, acute changes in the EKG are characteristic. However, in 20-50% of patients the EKG is non-diagnostic (subendocardial MI, LBBB, WPW, LVH). Furthermore, only 25-50% of old myocardial infarctions can be detected by EKG.

    c. Enzymes - in patients with a positive history for acute transmural MI and Q waves on EKG, SGOT, LDH and CPK-MB are elevated virtually all the time (94%, 100%, 100%). However, in patients with a history suggestive of an MI and with persistent ST-T wave changes (>24 hours), elevation of these enzymes is not as frequent (63%, 71%, 84%).

    d. Other Diagnostic Tests - echocardiography, nuclear radiology and cardiac catheterization are useful for detection of wall motion abnormalities and evaluation of ventricular function. These are discussed in the last section.

3. <u>Prognosis</u>. For the past 20 years, the annual mortality following myocardial infarction has been 5-8%. The acute in-hospital mortality is 10-40%. Following infarction, short-term and long-term prognoses are most significantly affected by:

    a. The degree of ventricular dysfunction following infarction.
       Highest risk: CHF symptoms, EF <.40, dyssynergy

    b. The site of infarction/extent of disease.
       Highest risk: anterior wall infarct, diffuse 3-vessel,
                    left-main disease

    c. The type of post-infarction dysrhythmias and conduction disturbances.

        Highest risk: fascicular block, complete heart block, serious ventricular dysrhythmias

4. Perioperative Risk.

PREVIOUS STUDIES

	1962 (Knapp)	1964 (Tompkins)	1972 (Tarhan)	1978 (Steen)	1978 (Goldman)	TOTAL (Avg)
Patients Studied	8,984	12,712	32,877	73,321	1,001	128,895
Previous MI	427	658	422	587	131	2,225
Reinfarction %	6.1	6.5	6.5	6.1	13.7(?)	6.8
Reinfarction Mortality %	58	70	54	69	67	65
% Reinfarction:						
0-3 months	100			37	27	
		55				36
3-6 months	100			16	11	

Previous studies have demonstrated that in patients with prior infarction: (1) the overall risk of reinfarction is 6-7% (vs <1% without previous MI); (2) with recent infarction (within 6 months), the risk of reinfarction is high (36 to 100%); (3) mortality with reinfarction is high (54 to 70%); and (4) the statistics have not changed over the previous two decades. However, a recent study has found significantly reduced six-month reinfarction rates (5%) and mortality (2%) when aggressive monitoring and therapy are used. These results have significant implication, and certainly warrant independent verification.

Given a patient with a recent infarction, what risk factors place that patient at highest risk?

Preoperative Risk Factors

  History: recent MI (<6 months), crescendo angina
Physical: hypertension, CHF
     EKG: Q waves, BBB, CHB, LVH (strain), ventricular dysrhythmia
     CXR: cardiomegaly, CHF
    Cath: 2,3-vessel disease, left-main disease, EF<50%, valve disease

In addition to these preoperative factors, the intraoperative factors associated with highest risk are: (1) surgery involving the great vessels, thorax, or upper abdomen; (2) emergency surgery; and (3) the degree and duration of intraoperative hypotension.

THE SIGNIFICANCE OF VENTRICULAR DYSFUNCTION IN CAD

1. **Incidence.** Approximately 700,000 patients die each year from CAD and its complications. With acute myocardial infarction, death usually results from ventricular dysrhythmias or failure. It appears that the mortality from dysrhythmias has been reduced by EKG monitoring and aggressive therapy. However, mortality from failure remains alarmingly high.

2. **Detection.** Quantitated ventriculography, nuclear cardiology and echocardiography provide sensitive measures of ventricular function: ejection fraction, wall motion, and myocardial compliance. The sensitivity of these is summarized by the following.

Measure	Abnormality first appears with:
Ejection Fraction	1,2-vessel disease (without MI)
Wall Motion (Dyssynergy)	3-vessel disease (without MI)
Compliance	MI
Cardiac Output	MI + 3-vessel disease
End Diastolic Pressure	MI + 3-vessel disease

3. **Prognosis.** In patients with acute or chronic CAD, the degree of left ventricular dysfunction is of major prognostic importance. Ejection fraction and dyssynergy appear to be the best prognostic indicators of short and long term survival. One year mortality is significantly higher (30%) in patients with ejection fractions <40%. In patients with three-vessel disease and EF<50%, the two year mortality is 36% (vs 12% with EF>50%). With single-vessel disease, patients with markedly abnormal wall motion have a five year mortality of 60% (vs 10% with normal wall motion). With three-vessel disease, the mortality is 90% (vs 35% with normal wall motion).

4. <u>Perioperative Risk</u>. In patients with manifest symptoms and
signs of left ventricular failure, the perioperative morbidity and
mortality are markedly increased. Preoperative assessment is relatively
straightforward. However, for the asymptomatic patient with CAD,
assessment of the risk of ventricular failure is more difficult. In
patients with CAD undergoing non-cardiac surgery, there are no
significant data. In patients undergoing myocardial revascularization,
the studies indicate that of all the preoperative screening data
(routine, EKG, and catheterization), ejection fraction and degree of
dyssynergy are the best predictors of left and right ventricular
dysfunction during the intraoperative and postoperative periods.
Furthermore, studies of short and long-term survival following cardiac
surgery have demonstrated that the preoperative LV ejection fraction is
the most useful prognostic guide compared with such measures as cardiac
output and end-diastolic pressure.

PREOPERATIVE ASSESSMENT: ADDITIONAL INFORMATION

The preoperative screening data most relevant to the assessment of
dysrhythmias, infarction and dysfunction are discussed above. In
addition, the following appear to be informative and prognostic.

History

1. Anginal pattern - stable vs unstable vs variant
                    - stress response, exercise tolerance
2. Dysrhythmia/failure symptoms with stress and effort.
3. Medication compliance (nitrates, beta blockers, Ca^{++} channel
blockers)

The history is the focal point of the assessment. However, there does
not appear to be a consistent relationship between the historical
features of angina (location, duration, precipitation) and the extent of
vessel involvement.

<u>Physical Examination</u>. On cardiac exam, the significance of the
following four findings is noteworthy.

1. Displaced PMI: Cardiomegaly - usually indicates an EF <.50 and
   places the patient at increased risk.

2. Precordial systolic bulge: Wall motion abnormality - usually indicates a prior MI or acute ischemia.

3. S_3: Increased LVEDP - usually indicates extensive MI.

4. S_4: Decreased LV compliance - usually indicates a prior MI or ischemia.

Chest X-Ray. In with CAD, cardiomegaly (cardiothoracic ratio >.50) is predictive of poor ventricular function (EF<.50) in approximately 70% of patients. Other changes (increased LV volume, increased total heart volume) are equally predictive.

EKG (resting). Positive Findings: The EKG is a reliable predictor of CAD only when: 1) significant Q waves are present, or 2) ST changes occur with spontaneous angina (stable, unstable or variant. Other findings on the EKG (ST-T wave changes, LBBB, LVH) are non-specific.

Negative Findings: A normal EKG does not preclude CAD. In 25-50% of patients with CAD the resting EKG is normal. However, it is rarely normal in the patient with significant left ventricular dyssynergy.

EKG (vector). Vectorcardiography is useful in depicting infarction patterns where the scalar EKG is equivocal. There is also evidence that selected abnormal vector patterns are indicative of severe abnormality of left ventricular function.

EKG (ambulatory-Holter). Compared with other methods of EKG monitoring, ambulatory monitoring significantly increases the yield of dysrhythmias. However, stress-response dysrhythmias may be missed. The yield of ST segment changes is also increased, and a good correlation exists between ST depression occurring during normal activity and angiographic findings. However, the artifact problem is significant, and affects the reliability of ST interpretation.

EKG (stress-testing). For dysrhythmia detection, the "exercise EKG (EEKG)" increases the yield of PVCs threefold (over the rest EKG) and eightfold for repetitive forms of ventricular dysrhythmias. Approximately 52% of patients with CAD exhibit PVCs on EEKG. The dysrhythmias usually occur not only at peak exercise, but also during the initial 3 minutes of recovery. In fact, ventricular fibrillation is most likely to occur during recovery.

For ischemia detection, the EEKG is informative if (1) the ST change is significant (> 2 mm); or (2) symptoms or hypotension occur with the ST change; or (3) the changes occur during the early testing period. Without these changes, it appears that exercise stress testing does not significantly improve diagnostic capability.

Echocardiography. One dimensional (M-mode) and two dimensional (2D) echocardiography are safe and non-invasive techniques used in CAD primarily for assessing left ventricular wall motion and function (LV volumes, ejection fraction). They have also been used for detection of left-main stenosis, LV aneurysms, septal rupture, papillary muscle abnormality and mural thrombus formation.

Wall Motion

1. M-mode echocardiography is not satisfactory. Although 1-2 mm sensitivity can be achieved, the beam is narrow (one dimensional) and only the basal LV is viewed.

2. 2D echocardiography is useful and reasonably accurate in 80-90% of patients with CAD. 2D wall motion abnormalities correlate well with the location and extent of acute MI scarring (post-mortem:dogs). Comparison with angiography demonstrates good correlation (84-97%), specificity (84%), and sensitivity (95%). Limitations include: 1) the technique varies from laboratory to laboratory; 2) technical difficulties (COPD, anatomic abnormalities) limit use; 3) multiple cross-sectional views are necessary; and 4) inferior-posterior dyssynergy is more difficult to detect (vs anterior).

Left Ventricular Function

1. M-mode echocardiography is inaccurate when dyssynergy is present. LV function is assessed by measuring the internal diameter of the LV along the beam at end-diastole ($LVID_d$) and end-systole ($LVID_s$). $LVID_d$ is accurate with or without dyssynergy. $LVID_s$, in the presence of dyssynergy, is inaccurate. Thus, estimates of ESV, SV, CO and EF may be inaccurate.

2. 2D echocardiography provides useful information if multiple cross-sections (> 2) are used. 2D ejection fraction correlates well with angiographic ejection fraction (.78 to .94). However, 2D left ventricular volumes consistently underestimate angiographic volumes by 30%, especially when less than 4 cross-sections are used. Thus, stroke volumes and cardiac outputs are underestimated. Estimates of ejection

fraction are more accurate because of cancellation of errors. However, 3 or more cross-sections should be used for accurate estimation of ejection fraction.

Nuclear Cardiology. Radioisotope imaging for detection of myocardial infarction and quantitation of ventricular function is safe and relatively non-invasive.

Myocardial Infarction. Use of radioisotope imaging for detection of myocardial infarction is useful when conventional methods (symptoms, EKG, enzymes) are equivocal or untimely (LBBB, WPW, <6 hours or >48 hours post-MI). Two different techniques are used: "hot spot" and "cold spot" imaging.

	"Hot Spot" Imaging	"Cold Spot" Imaging
Radionuclide	Technetium 99m-pyrophosphate	Thallium-201
Uptake by	Infarcted tissue	Normal tissue (normal perfusion and metabolism)
Positive with	Acute MI (>5 gm infarct)	Acute MI (>5 gm infarct) Old MI Ischemia
Timing: Earliest positive test	12-16 hours (post MI)	Immediately
Most sensitive	48-72 hours	<24 hours
Other uses	RV MI Subendocardial MI Infarct size (±)	Chamber size LVH, RVH, ASH Stress testing

Left Ventricular Function. Two techniques are used: first pass radionuclide angiography and gated cardiac blood pool.

	First-Pass	Gated-Pool
Radionuclide	Any technetium (99m) labelled pharmaceutical	Technetium (99m) labelled albumin or RBC
Type of technique	Transient (30 seconds) Multiple injections/hour	Steady state (6 hrs) Single injection/hr
EF correlation with angiography	>.90	>.90
Uses	LVEF Exercise testing Dyskinesis RVEF Intracardiac shunt	LVEF Exercise testing Dyskinesis
Geometric assumptions	None	Several

Cardiac Catheterization. Coronary angiography and ventriculography are the "gold standards" for definition of coronary anatomy and quantitation of ventricular function. In these regards, no other techniques are as accurate or informative.

Procedure

1. The catheter is advanced retrograde: peripheral artery to left ventricle.

2. Pressure measurements (systemic, ventricular, atrial) are made.

3. Ventriculography (single-plane or bi-plane) is performed using a highly osmotic contrast dye (10-18 ml/sec over 3-4 seconds).

4. Left ventricular volumes are measured (area-length method).

5. Segmental wall motion is quantitated (using hemiaxial shortening, segmental ejection fraction or percent asynergic segments).

6. Pressure measurements are repeated.

7. Selective coronary angiography is performed.

Information

Ventricular Function Data:

1) Ejection Fraction (most important)
2) Dyssynergy
3) Stroke Work
4) End-systolic Volume
5) End-diastolic Volume
6) Change in End-diastolic Pressure
   (dye)
7) Cardiac Output
8) End-diastolic Pressure

Angiographic Data:

1) Number and degree of vessel
   involvement
2) Presence of left-main
   (equivalent) disease –
   especially with a high grade
   right coronary lesion or a
   left-dominant circulation

REFERENCES

Background

1. Kannel WB, McGee D, Gordon T: A general cardiovascular risk
   profile: The Framingham Study. Am J Cardiol 38:46, 1976.
2. Gorleri R: Coronary Artery Disease. WB Saunders, Philadelphia,
   1976.
3. Cohn PF: Diagnosis and Therapy of Coronary Artery Disease. Little,
   Brown and Co., Boston, 1979.

Dysrhythmia

4. Ruberman LD, Weinblatt E, Goldberg JE et al: Ventricular premature
   beats and mortality after myocardial infarction. N Engl J Med
   279:759, 1977.
5. Jelinek MV, Lown B: Exercise stress testing for exposure of cardiac
   arrhythmia. Prog Cardiovasc Dis 26:497, 1974.
6. Angelini P, Feldman MI, Lufschanowski R et al: Cardiac arrhythmias
   during and after heart surgery. Prog Cardiovasc Dis 16:469, 1974.

Myocardial Infarction

7. Tarhan S, Moffitt EA, Taylor WF et al: Myocardial infarction after
   general anesthesia. JAMA 220:1451, 1972.
8. Goldman L, Caldera DL, Nussbaum SB et al: Multifactorial index of
   cardiac risk in noncardiac surgical procedures. N Engl J Med
   297:845, 1977.
9. Rao TLK, El-Etra A: Myocardial reinfarction following anesthesia
   in patients with recent infarctions. Anesth Analg 60:271, 1981.

Ventricular Dysfunction

10. Moraski RE, Russell RO, Smith M et al: Left ventricular function
     in patients with and without myocardial infarction and one, two,
     or three vessel coronary artery disease. Am J Cardiol 35:1, 1975.
11. Cohn PF, Gorlin R, Cohn LH et al: Left ventricular ejection
     fraction as a prognostic guide in surgical treatment of coronary
     and valvular heart disease. Am J Cardiol 34:136, 1979.
12. Mangano DT, Van Dyke DC, Ellis RJ: The effect of increasing
     preload on ventricular output and ejection in man: Limitations
     of the Frank-Starling mechanism. Circulation 62:535, 1980.

Assessment

13. Proudfit WL, Shirey EK, Sones FM: Selective cine coronary
     arteriography: Correlation with clinical findings in 1,000
     patients. Circulation 33:901, 1966.
14. Borer JS, Brensike JF, Redwood DR et al: Limitations of the
     electrocardiographic response to exercise in predicting coronary
     artery disease. N Engl J Med 293:367, 1975.
15. Reeder GS, Seward JB, Tajik AJ: The role of two-dimensional
     echocardiography in coronary artery disease. Mayo Clin Proc
     57:247, 1982.
16. Folland ED, Hamilton GW, Larson SM et al: The radionuclide
     ejection fraction: A comparison of three radionuclide techniques
     with contrast angiography. J Nucl Med 18:1159, 1977.
17. Mangano DT: Preoperative assessment of cardiac catheterization
     data: Which parameters are most important? Anesthesiology
     53:S106, 1980.

PREOPERATIVE EVALUATION OF THE PATIENT WITH CONGENITAL HEART DISEASE

ALVIN HACKEL, M.D.

The development of methods to diagnose and correct surgically congenital cardiac lesions is one of the most exciting chapters in recent medical history. Surgical procedures have been developed for the complete correction of many of the congenital cardiac lesions. Palliative procedures exist for others. The major challenge remains in the area of the hypoplastic heart syndrome and the medical treatment of pulmonary hypertension

Anesthesiologists have responded positively to the surgeons' challenge to develop methods for operating room anesthesia and post-operative intensive care for these severely ill patients.

The cardiovascular abnormalities requiring surgery in infancy and childhood are different than those of adults. Whereas adult cardiovascular surgery is mainly the treatment of coronary artery disease and/or left-sided valvular abnormalities, pediatric cardiac surgery is concerned with the treatment of congenital, rheumatic, and endocardial heart disease. In recent years, the rheumatic and endocardial lesions have decreased in frequency, leaving the congenital lesions as the most common concern.

Evaluation of the cardiovascular and pulmonary status depends on the type of cardiac pathology present. In order to predict the effect of anesthesia on the patient, a summation analysis of the effects of the anatomic abnormalities on the cardiovascular physiology is needed. The disease complex may involve a single anatomical shunt (eg., an atrial or ventricular septal defect) or a complex of abnormalities (eg., transposition of the great vessels with pulmonic stenosis and a ventricular septal defect).

The basic questions are (1) is a cyanotic (right-to-left) shunt or a non-cyanotic (left-to-right) shunt present? (2) what is the pulmonary blood flow and the pulmonary vascular resistance? (3) can the pulmonary vascular resistance be decreased by altering pulmonary blood flow? (4) will changing systemic or pulmonary vascular resistance effect the balance of systemic and pulmonary blood flow (the degree of shunting) and (5) has congestive heart failure, if present, been controlled by medical therapy?

At birth, the circulation goes through a "transitional" period changing from a fetal to an adult pattern. As the lungs are expanded, the pulmonary vascular resistance (PVR) falls and right-to-left shunts through the patent foramen ovale and the patent ductus arteriosus end. A number of physiologic factors can effect the pulmonary vascular resistance in a negative manner and prevent the anticipated drop in the PVR. The most important factors are hypoxia, acidosis, hypo- and hypervolemia, and hypothermia.

The blood volume of the neonate is difficult to measure and appears to have a wide variance around an approximate normal value of 90-100 ml/kg. Infants hypovolemic at birth are peripherally vasoconstricted with pale skin or "geographic mottling". The blood pressure should be taken but it may be misleading as the vasoconstriction will "protect" the blood pressure and lead to a falsely high value.

Neonates are poikilotherms with little ability to control their body temperature. They try to do so by increasing blood flow through areas of the body with deposits of "brown fat" and by peripheral vasoconstriction. There is increased oxygen consumption and decreased perfusion to the skin and other peripheral tissues resulting in metabolic acidosis. Since these mechanisms are very ineffective, these infants also cool off rapidly despite their efforts to stay warm. Our research and that of others indicates hypothermia in the distressed neonate (who later requires critical care transport to a regional care facility) is associated with a markedly increased mortality rate.

In addition to the disease entities, there are also physiologic differences between pediatric and adult cardiac patients. Of particular interest are the variations of cardiac output, heart rate, and blood pressure with age. A higher metabolic rate leads to an increased heart rate in the neonate and child. Cardiac output increases and heart rate decreases with age (Figure 1). Arterial pressure, on

16

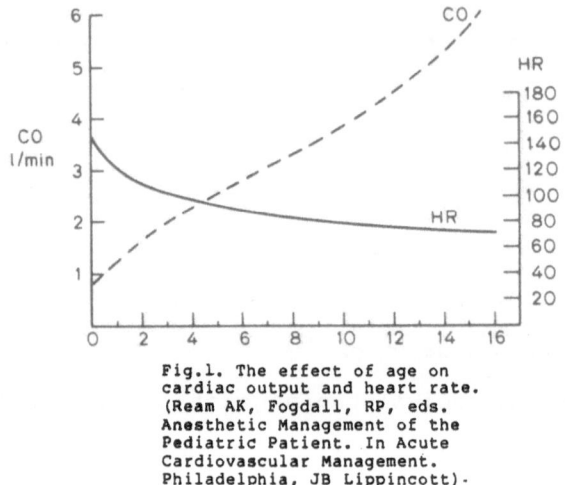

Fig.1. The effect of age on
cardiac output and heart rate.
(Ream AK, Fogdall, RP, eds.
Anesthetic Management of the
Pediatric Patient. In Acute
Cardiovascular Management.
Philadelphia, JB Lippincott).

the other hand, increases with age (Figure 2). The blood
volume as a fraction of body mass changes in the first two
years, gradually decreasing from 8.5 to 10 percent of body
weight at birth to 7 percent at two years of age.

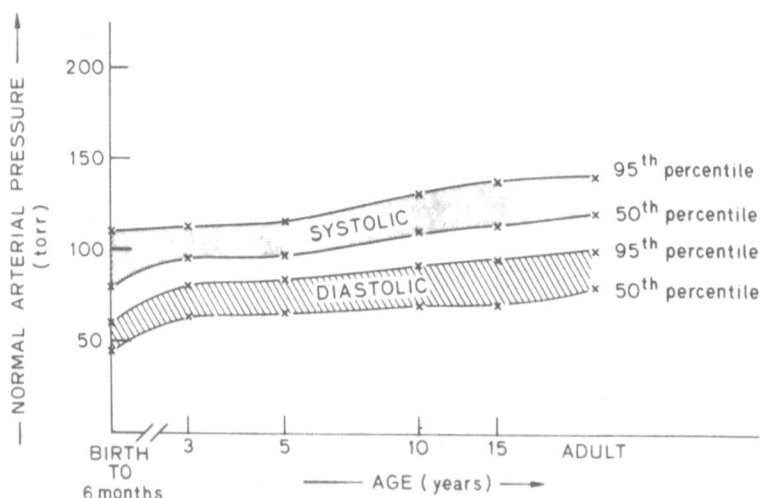

Fig.2. Arterial pressure norms versus age. (Ream AK,
Fogdall, RP, eds. Anesthetic Management of the Pediatric
Patient. In Acute Cardiovascular Management. Philadelphia,
JB Lippincott)

Hemoglobin and hematocrit changes with age are shown in Table 1. The red cell mass/blood volume ratio changes as fetal hemoglobin is replaced by adult hemoglobin in the first six months of life. This process of replacement leads to a significant shift in hemoglobin saturation versus pO_2 (Figure 3).

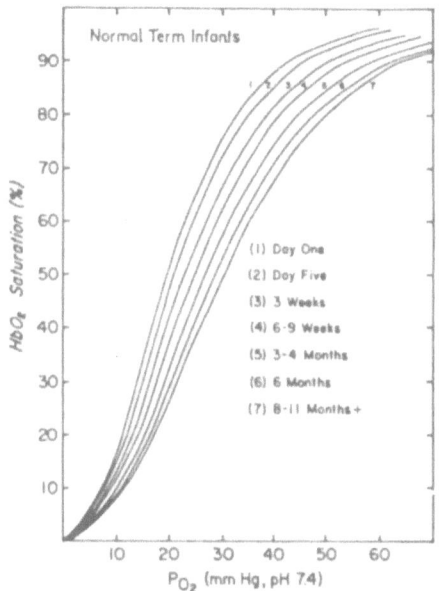

Fig. 3. Hemoglobin saturation versus arterial PO_2 (Ream, AK, Fogdall, RP, eds. Anesthetic Management of the Pediatric Patient. In Acute Cardiovascular Management. Philadelphia, JB Lippincott)

Pediatric patients differ from adults in their psychological reactions to hospitalization, anesthesia, and surgery. They (and their parents) suffer from the chronic anxiety of a prolonged debilitating and restricting illness associated with a shortened life expectancy.

Although the studies are not definitive, anxiety may

contribute to a poor prognosis in these patients.

Table 1. Normal Blood Values of Infants and Children. (Ream, AK, Fogdall, RP, eds. Anesthetic Management of the Pediatric Patient. In Acute Cardiovascular Management. Philadelphia. JB Lippincott).

AGE	HEMOGLOBIN (g/dl)	HEMATOCRIT PRCV/100 ml (means)
Birth (cord values)	13.6–19.6	56.6
1 day	21.2	56.1
1 week	19.6	52.7
4 weeks	15.6	44.6
2 months	13.3	38.9
6 months	12.3	36.2
1 year	11.6	35.2
2 years	11.7	35.5
4 years	12.6	37.1
8 years	12.9	38.9
10–12 years	13.0	39.0

(Smith CH: Blood Diseases of Infancy and Childhood. ed 3, p 16. St. Louis. CV Mosby 1972)

The preoperative evaluation begins with a determination of the child's general state of health and then focuses on the cardiovascular and pulmonary systems. An evaluation of growth and development with emphasis on exercise response must be included. The anesthesiologist should look for evidence of congestive heart failure, hypoxia and/or cyanotic episodes. Unless the surgery is an emergency, the presence of an infection, usually upper respiratory disease, is an indication for delay. Psychological preparation of the patient and the family should begin long before the anesthesiologist meets the family. Because of the chronic state of stress, the preoperative visit cannot be completely effective in allaying anxiety, but with care and expressed confidence, reassurance can be provided. Nevertheless, a careful simple non-threatening explanation of the role of the anesthesiologist and the concepts of the anesthesia to be used should be presented by the anesthesiologist.

The decision to withhold oral feedings preoperatively is made on the same basis as for other pediatric patients undergoing surgery. For infants receiving oral feedings every three to four hours, the last feeding is withheld and the previous feeding is restricted to clear liquids. For children eating three meals a day, there should be a six hour NPO period.

With patients in congestive heart failure, fluid restriction must be managed carefully. These patients may be dehydrated as a result of their preoperative medical preparation. Further dehydration will enhance hypovolemia and further decrease peripheral perfusion increasing the risk of patient injury. If the environmental temperature is above normal, if there is a delay in the beginning of surgery, or if the patient has polycythemia, it may be necessary to administer intravenous fluids.

Bibliography:

1. Hackel A. Preoperative Evaluation in Pediatric Anesthesia, Gregory G (ed). Churchill Livingstone, 1983.

2. Rudolph AM. Congenital Diseases of the Heart. Chicago, Year Book Medical Publishers, 1974.

3. Smith RM. Anesthesia for infants and children. St. Louis, CV Mosby, 1980.

AUTONOMIC NERVOUS SYSTEM AND ANESTHETIC MANAGEMENT

K. C. WONG

INTRODUCTION

   The body has a voluntary and an involuntary nervous system. The voluntary nervous system is controlled through the cerebal cortex by conscious commands, while the involuntary nervous system exerts its actions through the hypothalmus and other reflex mechanisms. The involuntary or autonomic nervous system provides homeostasis for the body, consisting of the sympathetic nervous system that prepares the body for stress while the parasympathetic nervous system prevents the overreaction of the sympathetic nervous system. This review discusses the neural transmitters of the sympathetic and parasympathetic nervous system, and some drugs which modify the actions or interactions of these neurotransmitters. This information will also provide the foundation for discussion by other lecturers of this postgraduate course.

SYMPATHETIC AND PARASYMPATHIC NERVOUS SYSTEM

   The sympathetic nervous system operates through the thoracolumbar (T_1-L_2) nerves and the adrenal medulla while the parasympathetic nervous system operates through the cranial sacral nerves. A schematic representation of the autonomic nervous system is shown in Figure 1. Sympathetic stimulation produces diffused response while parasympathetic stimulation produces more discrete responses. It is germaine to point out that acetylcholine is the neurotransmitter for both the sympathetic (nicotinic effect) and the parasympathetic ganglion as well as the post-ganglionic parasympathetic (muscarinic effect) neuroeffector site. Furthermore the adrenal medulla behaves like a ganglion where acetylcholine from a preganglionic fiber may cause a release of catecholamines from the adrenal medulla from a preganglionic fiber. A summary of some organ response to the autonomic nervous system stimulation is shown in Table 1.

AUTONOMIC NERVOUS SYSTEM

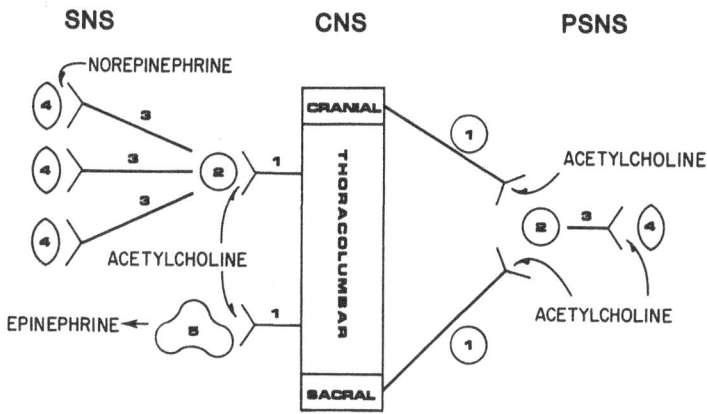

SNS **CNS** **PSNS**

1 PREGANGLIONIC FIBER
2 GANGLION
3 POSTGANGLIONIC
4 NEUROEFFECTOR SITE
5 ADRENAL GLAND

FIGURE 1. A schematic diagram showing that stimulation of the sympathetic nervous system (SNS) results in diffuse responses mediated at the post-ganglionic terminal by norepinephrine while stimulation of the parasympathetic nervous system (PSNS) results in more discrete responses because of a short post-ganglionic fiber in or near the affected organ. Note also that the adrenal medulla is, in effect, a functional sympathetic ganglion.

Table 1. Autonomic Nervous System Responses

	SNS	PSNS
Cardiovascular		
Heart rate	Increased	Decreased
Blood pressure	Increased	Decreased
Atria and ventricles	Increased contractility	Decreased contractility
Muscle B flow	Increased	Decreased
Skin B flow	Decreased	Increased
GI motility	Decreased	Increased
Bronchial muscles	Relaxation	Contraction
Eye		
Radial muscle, iris	Contraction	---
Sphincter muscle, iris	---	Contraction
Ciliary muscle	Relaxation	Contraction

The multiple distributions of acetylcholine as a neurotransmitter provide for some important and interesting drug interactions. Succinylcholine is structurally two acetylcholine molecules joined together at the acetyl groups. It is not surprising then that succinylcholine mimics many of the pharmacologic or physiologic actions of acetylcholine. In patients whose parasympathetic neuroeffector site is sufficiently blocked with an anti-cholinergic drug such as atropine, the administration of a cholinergic drug such as succinylcholine can produce an overt sympathetic stimulation by virtue of its stimulation of the sympathetic ganglion which is unmasked by the blockage of the post-ganglionic parasympathetic effector site. Succinylcholine has been reported to increase plasma catecholamine levels and cardiac arrhythmias in man. The use of edrophonium to treat paroxysmal atrial tachycardia has also precipitated cardiac arrest in the elderly patient. These findings emphasize the potential problems associated with the stimulation of acetylcholine receptors (sympathetic and parasympathetic) of the autonomic nervous system.

All general anesthetics directly or indirectly influence the autonomic nervous system or disturbing its balance. Drugs which control hypertension or angina can produce chemical sympathectomy. Other factors including disease, anesthetic technique and surgery add to the complexity of influences on the autonomic nervous system.

BIOSYNTHESIS AND DISPOSITION OF CATECHOLAMINES

The biosynthesis of catecholamines is shown in Table 2. Of importance in this scheme are the steps from the biosynthesis of dopamine to vanillylmandelic acid that may influence the anesthetic management. The sympathetic nerve terminal is the primary store of norepinephrine where stimulation of the sympathetic nervous system releases norepinephrine while catecholamine release from the adrenal medulla consists of 20% norepinephrine and 80% epinephrine. This ratio tends to reverse when an adrenal medullary tumor exists.

Table 2. Biosynthesis of Catecholamines

Substrate	Enzyme	Enzyme Inhibitors
Phenylalanine		
↓ ← Hydroxylase		
Tyrosine		
↓ ← Hydroxylase ←		α-methyl-p-tyrosine
Dopa		
↓ ← L-aromatic amino ← acid decarboxyase		α-methyldopa
Dopamine		
↓ ← Dopamine-β-hydroxylase ←		Disulfiram
Norepinephrine		
↓ ← Phenylthanolamine N-methyltransferase		
Epinephrine		
↓ ← COMT ←		Pyrogallal, Tropolone
Metanephrine		
← Monoamineoxidase ←		MAO inhibitors
↓		(Pargyline)
Vanillylmandelic acid		

Following a catecholamine receptor response, the most important mechanism by which the adrenergic response is terminated is the reuptake of the catecholamine into the sympathetic nerve terminal. Drugs which interfer with this neuronal reuptake mechanism will exaggerate adrenergic responses. Of lesser importance during anesthetic management are two other mechanisms which are responsible for the metabolism of the catecholamines. These are: 1) catechol-o-methyl transferase, a serum enzyme which promotes the addition of a methyl group to the catechol and 2) monoamine oxidase, an intraneuronal mitochondrial enzyme that promotes oxidative deamination of the catecholamines. Both mechanisms operate to maintain appropriate levels of catecholamines for the sympathetic nervous system. Catechol-o-methyl transferase has not been shown to be clinically important but inhibition of monoamine oxidase can produce serious exaggerated sympathetic response by virtue of the fact that a greater amount of catecholamine may be released from the nerve terminal during stimulation when the enzyme is inhibited by monoamine oxidase inhibitors.

DRUGS THAT EXAGGERATE SYMPATHETIC RESPONSES

1. Cocaine - Cocaine is a time honored local anesthetic and a potent
    vasoconstrictor. It is still a drug that is widely used among
    ENT and plastic surgery for hemostasis. Since cocaine inhibits
    neuronal reuptake of catecholamines, the peripheral sympathetic
    response is severely exaggerated. This is especially true when
    a combination of cocaine and epinephrine is used for hemostasis
    during halothane anesthesia. Hypertension, tachycardia and ven-
    tricular arrhythmias are common when this combination is used.
    Hypercarbia further exaggerates this sympathetic response.
    Effective treatment is adequate ventilation to eliminate excessive
    carbon dioxide with the administration of xylocaine or propranolol.
2. Imipramine - Imipramine is a tricyclic antidepressant which also
    inhibits the reuptake of catecholamines into the adrenergic nerve
    terminal. Imipramine has been shown to reduce ventricular arrhyth-
    mic threshold to epinephrine in dogs and in man it has been shown
    to interact with pancuronium to produce tachycardia and hyperten-
    sion. Halothane tends to potentiate while enflurane reduces the
    imipramine-pancuronium interaction on the sympathetic nervous
    system. Isoflurane similar to enflurane will also reduce the
    exaggerated sympathetic response of pancuronium and imipramine
    interaction.
3. Monoamine Oxidase Inhibitors - Although monoamine oxidase inhibi-
    tors have been largely replaced by tricyclic antidepressants, it
    is not uncommon to still see the use of MAO inhibitors in combina-
    tion with tricyclic antidepressants for treatment of psychiatric
    disorders. Pharmacologically, monoamine oxidase inhibitors may
    be present in the body for a short time but they produce irrever-
    sible inhibition of the intraneuronal enzyme. Regeneration of
    monoamine oxidase may take several weeks following the withdrawal
    of the drug therapy. There are no firm data to support the neces-
    sity for the withdrawal of monoamine oxidase inhibitors before
    surgery, however, early clinical experience of the 1950's and early
    1960's suggest that patients who are under the influence of mono-
    amine oxidase inhibitors tend to be hemodynamically unstable
    during general anesthesia. Therefore, there is still the general

belief that monoamine oxidase inhibitors should be withdrawn for at least two weeks prior to subjecting the patient to a general anesthetic.

It is important to realize that the advent of invasive monitors have greatly increased the ability to better assess the patient intraoperatively than was possible in the past. In the past decade emergency situations have dictated the author to provide anesthesia for patients who are on monoamine oxidase inhibitors for general anesthesia. The use of narcotic-nitrous oxide-oxygen-relaxant anesthesia regimen with a continuous monitoring of arterial pressure and central venous pressure have allowed reasonable anesthetic management without morbidity. The only clinical problem encountered is the impression that these patients required larger doses of CNS depressants to maintain general anesthesia. This is not unreasonable since increasing the catecholamine levels in the central nervous system should antagonize the depressant effects of drugs to the central nervous system.

4. L-dopa - L-dopa is widely used for treatment of paralysis agitans (Parkinson's disease). The pathophysiology of the disease may be related to a deficiency of dopamine as a neurotransmitter in the basal ganglion of the brain. Although dopamine itself crosses the blood-brain barrier with difficulty, L-dopa can cross the blood-brain barrier where it is converted to dopamine in the central nervous system. L-dopa is also converted to dopamine in the peripheral nervous system to enhance beta-adrenergic stimulation and cardiac arrhythmias in association with halothane anesthesia. Droperidol, which blocks dopamine, can exacerbate the manifestations of paralysis agitans. Although much has been discussed about L-dopa, there has not been serious anesthetic problem associated with its use.

5. Nitrous Oxide - Nitrous oxide is commonly used as an adjunct to inhalational anesthetics or narcotics. Nitrous oxide by itself is an alpha-adrenergic stimulant. The combination of using nitrous oxide-oxygen-barbiturates with relaxants was the "balanced anesthesia technique" of the 50's where a great deal of success was achieved by the use of the combination. More recent studies have shown that nitrous oxide when added to other agents tends to

reduce the salutary effects of inhalational or intravenous agents, i.e. when nitrous oxide is added to inhalational agents it tends to increase the potential to epinephrine induced arrhythmias as well as decreasing the cardiac output and increasing peripheral resistance. The addition of nitrous oxide to inhalational agents and narcotics also tends to reduce myocardial contractility. Therefore, although nitrous oxide is a time honored adjunct to other potent anesthetic agents, one should be cautious of the undesirable effects obtained when it is added to these agents.

DRUGS THAT ANTAGONIZE SYMPATHETIC ACTIVITY

1. Propranolol - The mechanism of action of propranolol as an anti-hypertensive and anti-anginal agent is related to its blockade of beta-adrenergic stimulation to the heart thus producing hypotension and reducing myocardial work and inhibition of renin-aldosterone system. The side effects of this drug is also related to its primary beta-adrenergic blocking action which may produce exacerbation of asthma, congestive heart failure, bradycardia and atrial ventricular conduction block. The withdrawal of propranolol in the preoperative period in patients with severe hypertension and angina has precipitated myocardial infarction and/or hypertension. Continuation of propranolol in the preoperative period is generally recommended.

2. Reserpine and Guanethidine - These agents have been used as the anti-hypertensive drugs in the past but have generally been largely replaced by other adrenergic blockers or vasodilating agents. These drugs act to reduce intraneuronal catecholamines by blocking the reuptake (reserpine) or the release of catecholamines from the nerve terminal (guanethidine). The recommendation in the past has been to withdraw these drugs before surgery, however, this has not been found to be necessary in clinical practice today, largely due to improved intraoperative monitoring and better assessment of the patient's hemodynamics.

3. Clonidine - Clonidine or Catapres is a centrally acting sympatholytic antihypertensive agent that has a biphasic action. Peripherally clonidine produces alpha-adrenergic vasoconstriction followed by hypotension from inhibition of central sympathetic outflow.

Clonidine is most frequently used for renal hypertensive patients and has been used in combination with propranolol. The most serious side effect related to anesthesia is the acute rebound hypertension observed after sudden and complete withdrawal of the drug. Signs of sympathetic overactivity are seen within 8-36 hours following the last oral dose and elevation of serum and urinary catecholamines have been noted. Although there has been the recommendation to withdraw the drug gradually before surgery, this author believes that the withdrawal is unnecessary and fraught with danger of rebound hypertension. It is generally accepted that patients who require significant anti-hypertensive or anti-anginal drug should not be withdrawn from these drugs.

CALCIUM CHANNEL BLOCKERS

Calcium channel blockers, Nifedipine and verapamil, are becoming widely used for treatment of angina and cardiac arrhythmias, respectively. Since calcium is necessary for myocardial contractility, the blockade of calcium movement can reduce myocardial contractility. When calcium channel blockers are used in combination with propranolol, the combination can further enhance myocardial depression of conduction, automaticity as well as contractility. The data are not available as to the potentiation of these drugs with anesthetic depression, but it is reasonable to believe that these drugs will indeed potentiate anesthetic depression of the myocardium. Therefore, caution should be exercised when anesthetizing patients on such drugs.

MANAGEMENT OF PATIENTS ON ANTI-HYPERTENSIVE OR ANTI-ANGINAL DRUGS
IN THE PERIOPERATIVE PERIOD

It is the general belief that a patient requiring these drugs should not be withdrawn prior to an anesthetic management, but there are a number of useful suggestions that might be offered when anesthetizing such patients.

1. Patients who are on anti-hypertensive drugs have poorly functioning compensatory sympathetic reflexes and will be more volume dependent for cardiac output.
2. The above patients may need protection from parasympathetic reflexes such as abrupt postural changes or excessive intra-

abdominal manipulation.

3. Special attention should be paid to a smooth induction, avoiding abrupt changes in drug concentrations.

4. Careful and continuous fluid replacement is mandatory; prophylactic use of plasma expanders, crystalloids or blood may be needed.

5. Serum cations, especially potassium, is important for myocardial rhythm and contractility. Both hyper- or hypokalemia will tend to exaggerate cardiac arrhythmias in the anesthetized patient. Maintaining normal intraoperative acid-base chemistry is an important step toward reducing cardiac arrhythmias.

REFERENCES

1. Symposium: The autonomic nervous system. Anesthesiology, Vol 29, July-August 1968.
2. Wong KC: Sympathomimetic agents. In Drug Interaction in Anesthesia. NT Smith, RD Miller AN Corbascio (Eds). Philadelphia: Lea & Febiger, 1981, pp 55-82.
3. Gilman AG, Goodman LS, Gilman A (Eds): Drugs acting at synaptic and neuroeffector junctional sites. In The Pharmacological Basis of Therapeutics. Macmillan Publishing Co., 6th ed. 1980, pp 56-220.
4. Nigrovic V, McCullough LS, Wajskol A, Levin JA, Martin JT: Succinylcholine-induced increases in plasma catecholamine levels in humans. Anesth Analg 62:627-32, 1983.
5. Rao TLK, Shanmugam M: Succinylcholine administration - Another contraindication. Anesth Analg 58:61-2, 1979.

MANAGEMENT OF THE DIABETIC PATIENT - PREOPERATIVE, INTRAOPERATIVE (DURING BYPASS) AND POSTOPERATIVE

SIMON DE LANGE

Cardiac surgery is a stressful event. Although techniques are being developed which may considerably reduce or minimize the haemodynamic response to the intraoperative stress of surgery, the endocrine, metabolic response is less well controlled. The control that is effected is at best temporary for no anesthetic technique so far developed has more than partially mitigated the endocrine response to the massive stress of cardiopulmonary bypass and hypothermia. Once initiated the response will augment the increase in catabolism that normally occurs after major surgery.

The diabetic patient is ill-equiped to face this metabolic challenge. Insulin is the only anabolic hormone which can effectively counteract the severe catabolism incurred. The mismanagement or denial of insulin administration can lead to severe postoperative metabolic derangement which may be difficult to correct and may jeopardize survival.

The stress response - metabolic changes

During stress, substrates are mobilised from storage sites and other tissues and redistributed to central organs. These metabolic changes are mediated by the stress hormones especially the catecholamines, cortisol and glucagon. They induce a catabolic state and oppose the action of the anabolic hormone insulin.[1] Glucose production is increased due mainly to hepatic glycogenolysis and gluconeogenesis. In addition, the uptake of glucose in the peripheral tissues is impaired.[2] The resultant hyperglycaemia is proportional to the severity of the stress reaction.[3] Increases of circulating fatty acids, glycerol, pyrurate, lactate and 3-hydoxybutyrate occur.[4]

Insulin secretion is inhibited by elevated catecholamine levels intraoperatively. Following surgery insulin levels become elevated but there is glucose intolerance or so-called insulin resistance.[1]

Metabolic changes in the diabetic patient during stress

There is an inappropriate increase of the stress hormones with rapid increase of substrates. Under the influence of high glucagon levels there is excessive ketogenesis without adequate disposal of ketone bodies. Ketoacidosis occurs as well as acidaemia.

Hyperglycaemia without the inhibiting effect of insulin continues to increase. Loss of electrolytes also occurs with ensuing diuresis and hyperosmolality develops.

These metabolic changes during and after cardiac surgery may impair cardiac performance, precipitate arrhythmias, increase the incidence of venous thrombosis and myocardial infarction.

Diabetic patients are divided into two types:
Type I   : Insulin dependent; juvenile in onset; prone to ketoacidosis.
Type II   : Insulin independent; maturity onset; obese and relatively insensitive to insulin, not prone to ketoacidosis.
             Vascular disease common.

Type II diabetics may be managed by diet alone but sometimes require exogenous insulin. More frequently they are controlled with oral hypoglycaemic agents.

The sulphonylureas (Chlorpropamide, Tolbutamide)
These stimulate release of insulin from the B cells of the pancrease. They can cause hypoglycaemia. Chlorpropamide has a long plasma half life - 36 hrs which may extend to 200 hours in renal disease.[5] In addition it exerts an antidiuretic effect. Cardiac surgical patients should have shorter acting sulphonyl ureas (Glibenclamide, Tolbulamide) substituted for chlorpropamide at least three days preoperatively.

The biguanides (phenformin) may act by promoting the anaerobic metabolism of glucose but also inhibit hepatic lactate disposal and may precipitate lactic acidosis in poor perfusion states. They should not be used in cardiac patients. However, if present preoperatively surgery should be postponed 48 hours and insulin therapy or short-acting sulphonyl ureas commenced.

Insulin metabolism and administration
1. Insulin has a half life in plasma of 9 minutes.[5] iv boluses have a short effect unless very large.

2. Renal failure may prolong action. Although resorbed by the kidney insulin is cleared by renal and hepatic metabolism.[5]

3. Insulin receptors. These become saturated and exert maximal effect at moderate levels of circulating insulin. Small but continuously administered amounts will be just as effective as intermittant large bolus doses.

4. Continuous intravenous infusion of insulin is the best method of administration.
   a) Infusion pump 1-2 units insulin/hour. This technique has been used with good results postoperatively.[6] Resistant cases of hyperglycaemia are treated with an insulin infusion pump in our clinic postoperatively.
   b) Combined insulin and glucose infusion is recommended.[1] It is safe since if the glucose infusion stops so will the insulin administration.

There is a continuous level of circulatory insulin with added substrate.
Adsorption of insulin on plastic and glass may reduce available insulin by 10-20% but may be compensated for by discarding the first 25-50 ml solution.

5. Subcutaneous insulin may have a depot effect with unreliable absorption during poor perfusion states or hypothermia. Walts and coworkers have shown that in surgical patients arbitrary insulin regimens which advocate 1/3-1/2 normal daily insulin dose preoperatively fall short of their intended goals.[7]
   They also advise that the control of blood glucose during surgery should be individualised and depend on blood glucose levels determined periodically during surgery and postoperatively.

Monitoring insulin therapy

During cardiac surgery monitoring of blood glucose should occur 1-2 hourly for good management. Ideally there should be concomitant base excess and plasma potassium determination to gauge metabolic homeostasis and potassium flux. Postoperatively blood glucose determination should be performed 2-3 hourly initially then 3-4 hourly on the second postoperative day. Results should be readily and rapidly available for satisfactory management.

Reflectance meters (Eyetone, Hypocount)

For those who do not enjoy this service or would like supplementary determinations in the OR, use of Dextrostix with a reflectance meter may provide a suitable alternative. A recent assessment showed that this method gave good correlations with standard blood glucose measurements.[8] The determination is easy and the meters relatively cheap but proper training in their use is essential with frequent reference to standard methods to obtain accuracy.

Urine glucose monitoring as a basis for insulin therapy is totally unsatisfactory in the cardiac surgical patient. The tests are retrospective and do not indicate changes in renal threshold which may occur during surgery.

Aims in the Management of the Diabetic Cardiac Patient

Preoperative

1) Prescreen patient on presurgical visit so that oral hypoglycaemic therapy may be modified if necessary and poorly controlled patients may have insulin therapy optimized.
2) Admit diabetic patients 24-48 hours preoperatively. Insulin dependant diabetics should be stabilized on soluble insulin with blood glucose control. Early admission and stabilization may avoid prolonged hospitalisation postoperatively.
3) Diabetic patients should be first on the OR list.

Intraoperative
1) Intravenous insulin therapy in all diabetic patients.
2) Avoid metabolic derangement.
3) Compromise on the side of hyperglycaemia especially during cardiopulmonary bypass (CPB) and hypothermia.
4) Avoid dangerous hyperosmolar blood glucose levels above 33 mmol/litre (600 mg/dl).
5) Minimize stress during surgery.

Postoperative
1) Restore metabolic homeostasis gradually.

General
1) Avoid hypoglycaemia at all costs.
2) Always ensure that there are at least basal levels of insulin and substrate available so that ketoacidosis does not develop. Starvation management - no insulin, no hypolgycaemia (and no severe hyperglycaemia) must be abandoned.
3) Maintain nourishment (5-10% glucose solution).

Management regimens
Two excellent management regimes for general surgical patients have recently been published. Walts and his coworkers favour intermittent bolus doses of insulin based on glucose levels with good results.[7]
Alberti and Thomas give a continuous infusion of 10% glucose and insulin with added potassium.[1] Insulin administration is altered according to blood glucose determination by altering the insulin concentration in the glucose solution. This method provided good control during general surgery. However during cardiac surgery with rapidly fluctuating conditions we find tight control difficult to apply.

Preoperative management
Type I 1) Early admission and stabilization on soluble insulin.
2) Nil orally from midnight before surgery.
   Emergency glucose drink by bed.
   Light sedation, only if necessary.
3) No subcutaneous insulin on day of surgery.
4) 6:00 a.m. day of surgery, 500 ml 5% glucose infusion commenced containing one quarter of daily soluble insulin requirement dose. The infusion rate is maintained at 80 ml/hour.
5) If the patient is still on lente insulin, daily soluble insulin requirment is estimated: -Daily lente insulin units x 1.5 = daily soluble insulin units requirement.
6) Blood glucose is monitored on arrival in OR (8:00 a.m.) but at least 2 hourly after commencing infusion.
7) Blood glucose < 5.5 mmol/l (100 mg/dl): Glucose-insulin infusion stopped and 5% glucose infusion substuted.

8) Blood glucose > 15 mmol/1 (270 mg/dl) 5 units soluble insulin added to infusion.
9) Standard premedication is given.

Type II 1) Patients admitted 24 hours before surgery and adequacy of blood glucose control monitored. Surgery is postponed 48 hours in patients still on biguanides.
2) Light sedation and nil orally from midnight. Emergency glucose drink available.
3) No oral hypoglycaemic agent on day of surgery.
4) 6:00 a.m. day of surgery, 500 ml 5% glucose with 4-6 units of soluble insulin commenced. 500 ml of this solution is given 6 hourly. The magnitude of this dose of insulin is decided on the adequacy of preoperative diabetic control.
The same infusion rate is maintained throughout surgery and postoperatively.
5) Patients on chlorpropamide are not given insulin in the 5% glucose solution until after blood glucose has been monitored (8:00 a.m.).
6) Subsequent preoperative management is as for Type I.

Premedication and beta adrenergic blockers

It has been found that insulin treated diabetics were no more prone to hypoglycaemia or hypoglycaemic unconsciousness than matched diabetic controls.[9] They also do not affect rate of fall of the blood glucose concentraiton in insulin induced hypoglycaemia.[10]
We neither discontinue beta blocking drugs in diabetics on the day of surgery nor withhold premedication for fear of unrecognised hypoglycaemia. However standard premedication is given only when it is certain the patient is going to the OR.

Intraoperative management Type I + II

1) The 5% glucose/insulin infusion is maintained at 80 ml/hour throughout surgery including bypass using an infusion control device. It is maintained as an independent system. Blood glucose, base excess and potassium is monitored hourly. Potassium supplementation is given separately when required.
2) Before cardiopulmonary bypass (CPB)
   a. Blood glucose maintained between 5.5-15 mmol/1 (100-270 mg/dl).
   b. Blood glucose < 5.5 mmol/1 - 5% glucose infusion substituted for glucose/insulin.
   c. Blood glucose > 15 mmol/1 - 5 units soluble insulin added to glucose/insulin infusion.
3) CPB and post CPB
   a. Blood glucose maintained between 5.5-20 mmol/1 (100-360 mg/dl).
   b. Blood glucose > 20 mmol/1 - 5 units soluble insulin added to glucose/insulin infusion.
   c. Blood glucose < 5.5 mmol/1 - substitution of 5% glucose

for glucose/insulin infusion.

Fluid management intraoperatively
A. Electrolyte solution containing <u>no</u> lactate are given as required (eg. Ringers)
   Lactate stimulates gluconeogenesis and increases hyperglycaemia especially in diabetics.[1]
   No extra glucose containing solutions are given unless metabolically required.
B. Pumpprime.
   a. Contains 500 ml 5% glucose (20% of volume) routinely
   b. No lactate containing solutions.
   c. Extra volume supplied by non glucose containing solutions.
      This avoids reaching dangerous hyerosmolar blood glucose concentrations.

Postoperative management Type I + II
1. The 5% glucose/insulin infusion is maintained at 80 ml/hour. Extra volume required is given as 5% glucose solution. Blood glucose, base excess and potassium are monitored 2 hourly initially and later 4 hourly.
2. Blood glucose limit 5.5-20 mmol/l. This upper limit is countenanced for 4 hours postoperatively or until normothermia.
3. Maintained blood glucose > 20 mmol/l
   a. Glucose/insulin infusion stopped and 5% glucose solution substituted.
   b. Insulin by infusion pump at 2 units/hour.
   c. Hourly blood glucose.
   d. If blood sugar falls by 5 mmol/l per hour or greater infsuion pump stopped and 5% glucose only given until fall levelled off.
4. On returning to solid diet insulin dependent diabetics are recommenced on routine insulin regimes and short-acting oral hypoglycaemic drugs are restarted in Type II diabetics using them preoperatively.

Anesthetic techniques
Techniques which modify the stress hormone release in response to cardiac surgery are desirable. High dose opioid techniques have been shown to fulfil these criteria at least until CPB.[11-13] Furthermore, it has been shown that insulin release was not significantly altered during cardiac surgery using high-dose fentanyl or sufentanil.[11, 13]
Thus high dose opioid anesthesia may be appropriate for Type II diabetics.

Special points in diabetics
1) Blood transfusion (high lactate and pyruvate levels), corticosteroid therapy and obesity may all increase insulin demand.
2) Renal disease may be present limiting insulin metabolism.
3) Autonomic neuropathy may cause cardiovascular instability intra- and post operatively.

4) Well managed diabetics in the intraoperative and perioperative period of cardiac surgery will benefit from improved wound healing and be less susceptable to postoperative sepsis thus avoiding prolonged hospilisation.

References
1. Alberti KGMM, Thomas DJB
   The management of diabetes during surgery.
   Br. J. Anaesth. 51: 693-710, 1979

2. Haljamae H
   Quantitation of surgical stress by the use of blood and tissue glucose and glycolytic metabolite levels.
   Reg. Anesth. 7: 557-59, 1982

3. Traynor C, Hall GM
   Endocrine and metabolic changes during surgery: anaesthetic implications.
   Br. J. Anaesth. 53: 153-160, 1981

4. Kehlet H, Brandt MR, Prange Hansen A, Alberti KGMM
   Effect of epidural analgesia on metabolic profiles during and after surgery.
   Br. J. Surg. 66: 543-546, 1979

5. Larner J, Haynes RC Jr
   Insulin and oral hypoglycaemic drugs; glucagon. In: The Pharmacological Basis of Therapeutics. Fifth edition, eds. Goodman LS, Gilman A, New York, Maxmillan Publ. Co., 1975

6. Taitelmann U, Reece EA, Bessman AN
   Insulin in the management of the diabetic surgical patient. Continuous intravenous infusion versus subcutaneous administration.
   JAMA 237: 658-660, 1977

7. Walts LF, Miller J, Davidson MB, Brown J
   Perioperative management of diabetes mellitus.
   Anesthesiology 55: 104-109, 1981

8. Webb DJ, Lovesay JM, Ellis A, Knight AH
   Blood glucose monitors: a laboratory and patient assessment.
   Br. Med. J. 280: 362-364, 1980

9. Barnett AH, Leslie D, Watkins PJ
   Can insulin-treated diabetics be given beta adrenergic blocking drugs?
   Br. Med. J. 280: 976-978, 1980

10. Lager I, Blohme G, Smith U
    Effects of cardioselective and non-selective beta-
    blockade on the hypoglycaemic response in insulin-
    dependent diabetics.
    Lancet 458-462, 1979

11. Sebel PS, Bovill JG, Schellekens APM, Hawker CD
    Hormonal responses to high-dose fentanyl anaesthesia.
    Br. J. Anaesth. 53: 941-948, 1981

12. de Lange S, Stanley TH, Boscoe MJ, de Bruijn NP, Berman
    L, Greene O, Robertson D
    Catecholamines and cortisol responses to sufentanil-O_2
    and alfentanil-O_2 anaesthesia during coronary artery
    surgery.
    Can. Anaesth. Soc. J. 30: 248-254, 1983

13. Bovill JG, Sebel PS, Fiolet JWT, Touber JL, Kok K,
    Philbin DM
    The influence of sufentanil on endocrine and metabolic
    responses to cardiac surgery.
    Anesth. Analg. 62: 391-397, 1983

PREOPERATIVE HYPERTENSION

F.G. ESTAFANOUS, M.D.

Hypertension is a world health problem. In the United States, it is estimated that one of every six persons may have hypertension. Less than half of these people are diagnosed as hypertensives and only 20% of those diagnosed may be receiving treatment. Hypertension occurs mainly in the middle and older age groups in both sexes and is seen in more women than men (1).

With the popularity of oral contraceptives, it was found that hypertension may develop in up to 5% of women who have been taking these drugs (2) for more than five years. The incidence is higher in those who have been using these hormones for a longer time and is related to the amount of progesterone in such preparations.

Hypertension in young adults occurs usually as secondary hypertension (3). In children it is definitely related to weight and a familial tendency to hypertension (4). In the United States, blacks have a higher incidence of hypertension and increased mortality from hypertensive heart disease than whites (5,6). There is also a definite correlation between obesity and hypertension (7).

Forty to eighty percent of diabetics are hypertensive (8). The incidence of hypertensive heart disease is five times greater in diabetics than in non-diabetics, especially diabetics suffering from nephritis.

Hypertension and Coronary Artery Disease

The same national health surveys which estimated that 15% to 20% of the American population suffers from hypertension, also estimated that 50% of hypertensive men and 70% of hypertensive women suffer from coronary artery disease (9). However, a large number of these patients may be unaware of both diseases.

Hypertension, per se, is an important cause of coronary artery disease. Blood pressure level is directly related to the atherosclerotic changes in both the coronary and systemic circulation, and as hypertension causes left ventricular hypertrophy, it disturbs the balance between myocardial oxygen supply and demand. Every manifestation of coronary artery disease has a significant relationship to the levels of both systolic and diastolic blood pressures (10,11).

The frequency of angina and myocardial infarction is twice as high in hypertensives as in normotensives (12); not only is the frequency of coronary artery disease much higher in hypertensives, the prognosis is worse. Congestive heart failure is more frequent in the presence of arterial hypertension and causes a high mortality.

Coronary artery disease by itself can predispose to episodes of severe hypertension, such as those observed during acute myocardial ischemia.

POSSIBLE CAUSES OF HYPERTENSION

A. Essential Hypertension (80% to 85%)

No definite cause is identified; however, these factors have some correlation to the incidence of essential hypertension:

1. Heredity
2. Salt intake
3. Disturbance of renin/angiotensin system
4. Disturbance of sympathetic nervous system controls.

B. Secondary Hypertension (15% to 20%)

Possible causes can be identified:

Kidney Disease

1. Acute and chronic infection
2. Ischemia of renal tissue, e.g., renal artery stenosis, trauma
3. Congenital abnormalities, e.g., polycystic kidney
4. Connective and collagen disease, e.g., polyarteritis nodosa, disseminated lupus, etc.

Endocrine Disease

1. Hyperaldosteronism (Conn's syndrome)
2. Pheochromocytoma
3. Toxemia of pregnancy

Neurogenic Causes

1. Sympatho-adrenal hyperactivity, e.g., tetanus
2. Stimulation of sympathetic cardiovascular reflexes, e.g., postmyocardial revascularization hypertension (13)
3. Coarctation of the aorta.

Hypertension varies in degree and severity. Mortality and morbidity are heavily dependent on severity. The severity of essential hypertension has been classified as follows:

1. Borderline hypertension (150/90 to 165/100 mmHg): Mortality rate 1.4 to 2.7 times that of a normotensive population.

2. Mild hypertension (sustained diastolic pressures greater than 100 mmHg): Mortality rate approximately three times that of a normotensive population.

3. Moderate hypertension (diastolic pressures 105 to 115 mmHg): Mortality rate over three times that of normotensive population.

4. Severe hypertension (diastolic pressure greater than 115 mmHg): 25% of these patients, if untreated, develop severe complications within a short time after initial detection.

PATHOPHYSIOLOGIC MECHANISMS OF HYPERTENSION

Recently, Tarazi et al (14) classified hypertension according to the pathologic and hemodynamic changes affecting the choice of therapy.

1. Volume-dependent hypertension: This type responds more to diuretic therapy and is relatively resistant to even large doses of neural blocking agents.

2. Hypertension associated with hyperkinetic circulation: Responds more to beta blockers as they control tachycardia, although this is not always the case as reduction of pressure is not a single effect of decreased cardiac output.

3. High renin hypertension: Responds to drugs that reduce plasma renin activity, such as propranolol, clonidine, methyldopa, guanethidine and reserpine.

4. High peripheral resistance hypertension: This is the hallmark of established essential hypertension whether related to neural or humoral factors. Patients with high peripheral resistance and low cardiac output will respond favorably to peripheral vasodilators. However, if the cause of the increased hypertension is increased peripheral resistance, it is logical to use neural blocking agents other than beta blockers.

5. Diminished aortic distendability: This is found in the elderly, particularly those with long-standing hypertension. It is usually recognized by wide pulse pressure, greater than 2/3 or 3/4 of the diastolic pressure. These patients also have diminished baroreceptor sensitivity.

In such patients, a marked fall in systolic pressure is expected with minimal interference with hemodynamic parameters.

ANESTHESIA AND HYPERTENSION

It has been estimated that over two million anesthetics are administered annually to hypertensive patients in the United States. These patients are at special risk. As early as 1919, Sprague (15) reported a 30% mortality and in 1935, Hickman (16) reported an 11% mortality in hypertensive patients undergoing surgery. In 1946, Peet (17) reported a surgical mortality of 10% in patients undergoing thoracolumbar sympathectomy for treatment of hypertension. Prys-Roberts and colleagues studied many aspects of the hemodynamic changes in hypertensive patients during anesthesia and surgery, and emphasized the special risks of hypertension associated with coronary artery disease (12).

In the last decade, much progress has been made in the treatment of hypertension and management of anesthesia. Preoperatively, however, hypertensive patients are still at special risk. Among the many factors that cause these special risks are 1) cause and degree of hypertension; 2) interactions between the hypertensive medication and anesthetic agents; and 3) effect of anesthetic agents and muscle relaxants on both the myocardium and the peripheral circulation.

Preoperative Evaluation of the Hypertensive Patient

Preoperative evaluation of the hypertensive patient should emphasize the following:

1. Severity and duration of hypertension

2. Presence of a primary disease for which surgery may be scheduled as treatment for hypertension, such as coarctation of the aorta, renal stenosis, pheochromocytoma, etc.

3. The extent of target organ involvement and functional status of the heart, kidneys, coronary circulation, and peripheral circulation.

4. The predominant mechanism associated with hypertension.

5. The possible side effects of preoperative drug therapy; effects of continuing or discontinuing of such antihypertensive agents on management of anesthesia.

Frequently, patients are admitted to surgery without a history of hypertension but do have symptoms suggestive of a latent pheochromocytoma. A severe, unexplained hypertensive crisis provoked by the stress of surgery and anesthesia can endanger the patient's life (18-20).

The following findings are always suggestive of pheochromocytoma:

    Headache, palpitations, tachycardia, tremor

    Hypermetabolism without hyperthyroidism

    Symptomatic paroxysms of hypertension

    Short history of hypertension (less than two years)

    Hypertensive retinopathy.

The presence of any or all of these indicates further evaulation to diagnose or exclude the presence of a catecholamine-secreting tumor.

In patients receiving preoperative diuretic therapy, the serum potassium should be checked prior to surgery.

Special attention should be paid to the patient to reassure him and acquaint him with the nature of the surgical procedure, the set-up, what to expect before surgery and afterwards in the intensive care unit.

Strong premedication will help to minimize undesirable hypertensive episodes during transfer from his room to the surgical suite.

We routinely use transdermal sustained-release nitroglycerin as a component of premedication. It is valuable in the presence of coronary artery disease and it helps to minimize an undue rise in blood pressure prior to induction of anesthesia.

Preoperative Hypertensive Therapy

The question of discontinuation of antihypertensive treatment before anesthesia is a legacy of the early days when little was known about the mechanisms influencing blood pressure control and the pharmacology of drugs, and because of the widespread use of long-acting sympatholytic agents (22-25).

Reserpine and Guanethidine

These agents cause marked depletion of norepinephrine from sympathetic nerve endings with the following consequences during anesthesia and surgery: 1) an exaggerated reaction to inhalation anesthetic agents, such as halothane, which can cause myocardial depression and peripheral vasodilatation; 2) undue dependence of blood pressure levels on fluctuations of intravascular volume; such changes can be direct due to blood loss during surgery, or be an indirect effect of the muscle relaxants as they decrease the muscle tone and venous return; 3) marked sensitivity to catecholamine pressor agents. These effects explain the severe hypotension encountered during anesthesia and surgery and the

severe episodes of hypertension when sympathomimetic vasopressors are used
to counteract the drop in blood pressure (20-23).

These problems and the early impressions of Inderal led to recommendations to discontinue these drugs two weeks prior to surgery (24).
Now more is known regarding cardiovascular control mechanisms, the hazards
of hypertensive crises, and the mode of action of new antihypertensives,
which is quite different from the long-acting antihypertensive
sympatholytic agents (14).

Abrupt discontinuation of central alpha adrenergic stimulants such as
clonidine or beta blockers can lead to a hypersympathetic state. This is
a general syndrome consisting of tremors, restlessness, insomnia,
tachycardia, mild dilation of the pupils. In severe cases, particularly
in patients receiving clonidine and in patients taking beta blockers,
severe paroxysmal hypertension, anginal pains, and signs of myocardial ischemia and myocardial infarction may occur.

In fact, beta adrenergic blockers minimize hypertensive responses to
sympathetic stimulation and reduce the incidence of dysrhythmias and EKG
signs of ischemia (25). Currently, beta adrenergic blockers are used to
control heart rate and rise in blood pressure during anesthesia and
surgery. They are also used to protect the myocardium during anesthesia,
particularly during cardiac surgery.

Vasodilators and Other Antihypertensives

Most other antihypertensive agents are either vasodilators or short-
acting drugs that do not lead to the same degree of denervation hypersensitivity as agents that deplete peripheral nerve endings of catecholamine
or block autonomic ganglia. It is neither necessary nor useful to discontinue this medication before surgery. The converting enzyme inhibitors
have a large and rather safe record regarding discontinuance of therapy.
The blood pressure does not rebound, and in fact, will only slowly come
back to its original level so that the patient can take the last dose the
night before surgery and resume it within a couple of days without having
been subjected to the risk of undue elevation of blood pressure.

Calcium Entry Blockers:

Calcium entry blockers pose a special problem (26). In general,
these are short-acting agents, with effects that will not last beyond 24
hours (27). They are commonly viewed as pure myogenic vasodilators that

prevent blood vessel constriction by interfering with the movement of calcium in the muscle fibers. However, since they affect the final common
pathway of vasoconstriction, they might block response to sympathetic
nerve stimulation. Clinical reports warn of the possibility of significant hypotension during induction in patients receiving calcium channel blockers. However, recent studies found no correlation between serum
nifedipine levels and blood pressure changes during induction (28). This
is still an active area of research. It is difficult to be dogmatic about
the implications of calcium entry blockade in the choice of pressor agent
should hypotension prove to be a problem.

Diuretics

The only drugs for which one could see a rationale for discontinuance
before anesthesia are the diuretics. Because of the effect of diuretic
therapy on potassium levels, severe hypokalemia may cause serious ar-
rhythimas (29). Also, it would help us to understand the paradox that the
kidney is subjected to much less workload when the patient is
over-hydrated than when he is deprived of salt and water. It is our aim
to secure a good urinary flow following surgery because the hypertensive
patient going to surgery dehydrated is at greater risk of renal complications. Hence, it has been our custom to discontinue diuretics a day or
two before surgery. This leads to a rebound retention of fluid and the
patient can go through surgery with less likelihood of renal complications.

Finally, if a patient has been on some form of therapy, including
long-acting agents such as reserpine or guanethidine (particularly reserpine, which is still used extensively in some states and in some public
health programs), the main measures to remember are: 1) discontinuing the
drug a day or two before surgery would not alter the fact that the patient
is functionally sympathetically denervated; 2) in these cases, blood
volume control depends mainly on control of intravascular volume; and 3)
if the patient still needs vasopressors, one must remember the hypersensitivity to catecholamines and either use very small doses, or resort to
other vasoconstrictors.

Anesthesia and the Hypertensive Patient

Induction of anesthesia, is always accompanied by significant
hemodynamic changes. The magnitude of these changes depends on many factors such as a) preoperative disease and hemodynamic status; b) preopera-

tive drug therapy (22-23); c) the type of anesthetics and muscle relaxants used; d) sympathetic stimulation by laryngoscopy, endotracheal intubation, nasopharyngeal cannulations, etc. (30); e) initiation of positive pressure ventilation (31); and f) the experience of the practicing anesthesiologist. In this chapter, we can only allude to factors relevant to hypertensive patients, who will respond in an exaggerated manner to all of these variables and are more vulnerable to blood pressure changes.

Hemodynamic responses in hypertensives vary in each individual depending on type and degree of hypertension, hemodynamic changes of that particular hypertensive state such as hypovolemic or hypervolemic, hyperkinetic circulation, increased sympathetic tone, increased systemic vascular resistance, antihypertensive treatment, etc. (14). In view of all of these variables, the blood pressure can move to either direction, hypotension or hypertension. The risks of such changes are more profound in hypertensive patients who also suffer coronary artery insufficiency (32-33) or cerebrovascular disease. A rise in blood pressure, particularly if accompanied by tachycardia, will seriously increase myocardial oxygen consumption, whereas hypotension in a patient with partially occluded coronary vessels can seriously decrease myocardial blood flow. The net result is a high incidence of postoperative myocardial infarction.

In patients with cerebrovascular disease, extreme changes in blood pressure can cause cerebrovascular hemorrhages or cerebral ischemia and generalized encephalopathy. Indeed, the incidence of postoperative neurological and psychological complications, particularly in elderly patients, cannot be overemphasized (34). Therefore, every effort should be made to plan the management of anesthesia that produces minimum changes in blood pressure during induction.

Two questions deserve further discussion:

1. The need to initiate antihypertensive treatment prior to induction of anesthesia

One normally assumes that unless the patient is in hypertensive crisis prior to induction of anesthesia, there is no indication to start specific antihypertensive treatment. However, if a severely hypertensive patient must be operated upon immediately, such treatment may be indicated. The patient must be adequately monitored: right and left side filling pressures, cardiac output and systemic vascular resistance values should be available during such an emergency. Treatment should be

directed not only toward lowering the blood pressure, but also toward
maintaining positive myocardial oxygen supply/demand, prevention of ischemia, and maintaining adequate blood volume to minimize the possibility
of severe hypotension during induction.

2. Appropriate depth of anesthesia

Light planes of anesthesia during induction were considered ideal for
hypertensive patients (32). A strong argument against this approach, is
that light planes of anesthesia will not eliminate or decrease the
responses to sympathetic stimulation by laryngoscopy, intubation and
surgery. On the contrary, hypertensive reflexes may be exaggerated with
such light planes of anesthesia. Ideally, the patient should be adequately anesthetized and the cardiovascular responses to sympathetic
stimulation and blood pressure fluctuations should be minimal. In such
highly sensitive patients, all of these measures may not be achieved by
anesthetic agents or muscle relaxants alone, and adjuvant vasoactive drugs
such as vasopressors, vasodilators and beta blockers may be needed for
fine adjustment of the hemodynamic parameters.

Intravenous barbiturates produce marked changes in the arterial pressure of the hypertensive patient when doses are the same as those used in
the normotensive patient. Diazepam and narcotics cause an even more significant fall in blood pressure (33).

Narcotics: Years ago, Prys-Roberts and Foex reported that "Small
doses of fentanyl (3-4 mcg/kg) followed by a small dose of sodium pen-
tothal caused minimum hemodynamic changes in the hypertensive patient"
(32-33). This small dose of the drugs used, even in the presence of
strong premedication, will not produce the level of anesthesia that can
eliminate or even decrease sympathetic stimulation. In our experience
with relatively large doses of fentanyl (40-60 mcg/kg) as the sole induction agent, the hemodynamic changes during induction and intubation are
minimal and the incidence of hypotension is extremely rare. At this
point, we have to reemphasize that vasoactive cardiovascular drugs should
be available to immediately control unacceptable changes in blood pressure
and heart rate in either direction as they occur.

Inhalation Agents: In the hypertensive patient, halothane causes
lability of the blood pressure and lowers intraoperative systolic blood
pressure. These patients also require more frequent intraoperative fluids
and adrenergic agents (35). Nitrous oxide added to halothane, further

lowers the blood pressure and decreases cardiac output (36). In hypertensive rats, halothane anesthesia results in greater changes in distribution of blood flow as compared with enflurane and decreases blood flow to vital organs suggesting that the margin of safety is diminished.

Enflurane has more peripheral vascular effects than halothane and may cause a more profound drop in blood pressure in preoperatively hypertensive patients (37).

Maintenance of anesthesia by narcotics and nitrous oxide may be more satisfactory for the hypertensive patient (33). However, the experienced anesthesiologist will finely adjust the hemodynamic changes as needed by anesthetic or vasoactive agents.

Muscle Relaxants: Muscle relaxants are almost always a component of induction agents. The choice of muscle relaxant is another important factor in determining the magnitude of hemodynamic changes during induction. The ultimate hemodynamic changes during induction are the sum of the effects of both induction agent and muscle relaxant. In the literature, there are no meaningful studies concerning the hemodynamic effects of muscle relaxants on hypertensive patients. Nevertheless, we can postulate what these effects can be from reviewing the hemodynamic effects of the muscle relaxants. Pancuronium bromide increases heart rate, mean arterial pressure, pulmonary capillary wedge pressure, and may decrease systemic vascular resistance, whereas metocurine also increases heart rate and cardiac output but does not change the MAP or pulmonary capillary wedge pressure. On the other hand, d-tubocurarine decreases cardiac output, systemic vascular resistance and MAP. New muscle relaxants, such as Org NC 45 (38) or atracurium have fewer cardiovascular effects than pancuronium, metocurine or d-tubocurarine (39).

In the context of discussing muscle relaxants in the hypertensive patient, the use of preoperative ganglion-blocking therapy can potentiate the effect of non-depolarizing muscle relaxants (40). An antihypertensive agent capable of releasing acetylcholine can potentiate the effect of both depolarizing and polarizing muscle relaxants (41).

Intraoperative Monitoring of the Hypertensive Patient

Preoperative hypertension, with all the risks involved, is an indication for more comprehensive monitoring, particularly during induction of anesthesia and surgery. The extent of this monitoring should be tailored to the extent and duration of surgery. However, it is necessary to emphasize that many of the hypertensive patients undergoing major surgical procedures, particularly those having surgery of the abdominal aorta or carotid endarterectomy, have a high incidence of severe coronary artery disease.

For minor and short surgical procedures, noninvasive monitoring can be adequate. As a minimum requirement:

1. EKG, Lead V, should be continuously displayed. Signs of ischemia are detected in 90% of cases by Lead V, much more than any other single lead.

2. Frequent blood pressure measurements to detect early any significant blood pressure changes.

For major lengthy surgical procedures, invasive monitoring is preferable:

1. Arterial cannulation and continuous monitoring of both systolic and diastolic blood pressures; these indicate both myocardial oxygen consumption and coronary perfusion. This is preferable to a display of mean arterial pressure.

2. Pulmonary artery double lumen catheters: they will facilitate monitoring of right and left filling pressures and measurement of the cardiac output. Calculating systemic vascular resistance, pulmonary vascular resistance and other hemodynamic indices helps to reach a specific diagnosis for the causes of changes in either blood pressure or cardiac output. Such specific diagnosis will allow appropriate selection of vasoactive agents when required.

48

REFERENCES

1. Gordon T: Blood pressure of adults by age and sex, United States 1960-62. National Center for Health Statistics, PHS Publ. 1000, ser. 11, no 4, 1964.
2. Oral contraceptives and health: An interim report from the oral contraception study of the Royal College of General Practitioners. Pitman Medical, London, p 98, 1974.
3. Brest AN, Moyer JN: Diagnosis of hypertension, in The Heart, Arteries and Veins, 2nd ed., edited by JW Hurst and Logue RB, McGraw-Hill, New York, p 1070, 1970.
4. Platt R: Essential hypertension. Incidence, course and heridity. An Intern Med 55:1-11, 1961.
5. Moriyama IM, Krueger DE, Stamler J: Cardiovascular diseases in the United States, Harvard, Cambridge, Mass., p 124-125, 1971.
6. Gordon T: Blood pressure of adults by race and area, United States 1960-62. National Center for Health Statistics, PHS Publ. 1000, ser. 11, no. 5, 1964.
7. Tyroler HA, Heyden S, Hames CG: Weight and hypertension: Evans County studies of blacks and whites, in Ref. 2, p 177-201.
8. Christlieb AR: Diabetes and hypertensive vascular disease: Mechanisms and treatment. Am J Cardiol 32:592-606, 1973.
9. Hollander W: Hypertension, antihypertensive drugs and atherosclerosis. Circulation 48:1112-1127, 1973.
10. Kannel WB, Schwartz MJ, McNamara PM: Blood pressure and risk of coronary heart disease - The Framingham study. Dis Chest 56:43, 1969.
11. Inter-Society Commission for Heart Disease Resources. Arteriosclerosis Study Group and Epidemiology Study Group: Primary prevention of the atherosclerotic diseases. Circulation 44:A263, 1971.
12. Prys-Roberts C: Medical problems of surgical patients: Hypertension and ischaemic heart disease. Ann R Coll Surg Engl 58:465-472, 1976.
13. Estafanous FG, Tarazi RC, Viljoen JF, El Tawil MY: Systemic hypertension following myocardial revascularization. Am Heart J 85:732-738, 1973.
14. Tarazi RC: Hypertension, In, Current Therapy, 1977, ed. Conn HF, W.B. Saunders Co., Philadelphia, pp:205-221.
15. Sprague HB: The heart in surgery. An analysis of the results of surgery on cardiac patients during the past ten years at the Massachusetts General Hospital. Surg Gynecol Obstet 49:54-58, 1929.
16. Hickman J, Livingstone II, Davies ME: Archives of Surgery, 31:917-936, 1935.
17. Peet MM, Isberg EM: Surgical treatment of essential hypertension. JAMA 130:467-473, 1946.
18. Gifford RW: Evaluation of the hypertensive patient. Chest 64:336-40, 1973.
19. Gifford RW, Kvale WF, Maher FT, et al: Clinical features, diagnosis and treatment of pheochromocytoma: A review of 76 cases. Mayo Clin Proc 39:281-302, 1964.
20. Coakley CS, Alpert S, Boling JS: Circulatory responses during anesthesia of patients on rauwolfia therapy. JAMA 161:1143-44, 1956.
21. Ziegler CH, Lovette JB: Operative complications after therapy with reserpine and reserpine compounds. JAMA 176:916-919, 1961.
22. Munson WM, Jenicek JA: Effect of anesthetic agents in patients receiving reserpine therapy. Anesthesiology 23:741-745, 1962.
23. Katz RL, Weintraub HD, Papper EM: Anesthesia, surgery and rauwolfia. Anesthesiology 25:142-147, 1964.

24. Viljoen JF, Estafanous FG, Kellner GA: Propranolol and cardiać surgery. J Thorac Cardiovasc Surg 64:826-830, 1972.

25. Prys-Roberts C, Foex P, Biro GP, Roberts JG: Studies of anaesthesia in relation to hypertension. V: Adrenergic beta-receptor blockade. Br J Anaesth 45:671-680, 1973.

26. Reves JG, Kissin I, Lell WA, et al: Calcium entry blockers: Use and implications for anesthesiologists. Anesthesiology 57:504-518, 1982.

27. McAllister RG: Clinical pharmacokinetics of calcium channel antagonists. J Cardiovasc Pharmacol 4:S340-S345, 1982.

28. Reves JR, Barker S, Smith LR: Significance of nifedipine plasma levels and hemodynamic changes during anesthesia induction. Anesthesiology 59 (3):A41, 1983.

29. Scribner BH, Burnell JM: Symposium: Water and electrolytes, interpretation of serum potassium concentration. Metabolism 5:468-479, 1956.

30. Prys-Roberts C, Greene LT, Meloche R, Foex P: Studies of anaesthesia in relation to hypertension. II: Haemodynamic consequences of induction and endotracheal intubation. Br J Anaesth 43:531-545, 1971.

31. Foex P, Meloche R, Prys-Roberts C: Studies of anaesthesia in relation to hypertension. III: Pulmonary gas exchange during spontaneous ventilation. Br J Anaesth 43:644-661, 1971.

32. Prys-Roberts C, Meloche R: Management of anesthesia in patients with hypertension or ischemic heart disease. Int Anesthesiol Clin 18:1-23, 1980.

33. Foex P: Anesthesia for the hypertensive patient. Cleve Clin Q 48:63-67, 1981.

34. Breuer AC, Hanson MR, Furlan AJ, et al: Central nervous system complications of myocardial revascularization. A prospective analysis of 400 patients. (Abstr) Stroke 11:136, 1980.

35. Goldman L, Caldera DL: Risks of general anesthesia and elective operation in the hypertensive patient. Anesthesiology 50:285-292, 1979.

36. Prys-Roberts C, Foex P, Greene LT, et al: Studies of anaesthesia in relation to hypertension. IV: The effects of artifical ventilation on the circulation and pulmonary gas exchanges. Br J Anaesth 44:335-347, 1971

37. Miller ED, Jr., Beckman JJ, et al: Cardiovascular responses to anaesthetic agents in hypertension. Anesthesiology 59 (3):A50, 1983.

38. Booji LH, Edwards RP, Sohn YJ, et al: Cardiovascular and neuromuscular effects of Org NC 45, pancuronium, metocurine, and d-tubocurarine in dogs. Anesth Analg 59:26-30, 1980.

39. Sokoll MD, Gergis SD, Mahta M, Kemmotsu O, Rudd D: Haemodynamic effects of atracurium in surgical patients under nitrous oxide, oxygen and isoflurane anesthesia. Br J Anaesth 55:775, 1983.

40. Paton WD, Zaimis EJ: The methonium. Pharmacol Rev 4:219-253, 1952.

41. Boura AL, Green AF: The actions of bretylium: adrenergic neurone blocking and other effects. Br J Pharmacol 14:536-548, 1959.

CALCIUM ANTAGONISTS AND ANESTHESIA

J.G. REVES, M.D.

The purpose of this report is to update a previous, more detailed review of calcium entry blockers and the implications these drugs have on anesthesia practice.[1] In our previous paper we did not include diltiazem which has recently been released and whose pharmacology has been reviewed by McAuley and Schroeder.[2] A number of other excellent review articles pertinent to the subject have also appeared since our listing of pertinent papers.[3-11]

Calcium Antagonists

There are three structurally diverse calcium antagonists available at present (1983) in the United States: nifedipine (Procardia), verapamil (Isoptin, Calcan) and diltiazem (Cadiozem). Some of their pharmacologic characteristics are listed in Table I.

Table I.

PHARMACOLOGIC CHARACTERISTICS OF CALCIUM CHANNEL BLOCKERS

	NIFEDIPINE	VERAPAMIL	DILTIAZEM
Dosage			
oral	10-20 mg t.i.d.	80-160 mg t.i.d.	40-80 mg t.i.d.
i.v.	5-15 mcg/kg	150 mcg/kg	15-30 mcg/kg
Absorption			
oral (%)	> 90	> 90	> 90
bioaval (%)	65-70+	10-20	?
Onset Action			
oral (min)	< 20	< 30	< 30
subl (min)	3	-	-
i.v. (min)	1-3	1-3	1-3
Protein Binding (%)	90	90	80-85%
Elimination t½ (hr)	2-5*	2-7*	4-6
Active metabolites	no ?	yes	yes
Excretion			
renal (%)	80	70	35
fecal (%)	< 15	15	65

Where Bioaval = bioavailability, subl = sublingual, + nifedipine is light sensitive and should be protected from light, * = normal patients

Of interest to anesthesiologists is the elimination t½ or elimination half-life of the drugs since this gives an indication of the decrease of serum blood level after cessation of therapy. All have relatively short half-lives (about 4 hours). Also of interest is the fact that both verapamil and diltiazem have active metabolites; the half-lives of these compounds have not been fully evaluated.

Since calcium is essential in excitation contraction coupling of cardiac and vascular smooth muscle, it is not surprising that the primary pharmacologic effects of the calcium antagonists are hemodynamic. Indeed, these drugs are prescribed for the control of arrhythmias (verapamil and diltiazem) and classical and/or variant angina (nifedipine, verapamil and diltiazem) because of their electrophysiologic and cardiovascular effects. The calcium antagonists primarily cause vasodilation by "excitation uncoupling"[9] which means that cytosol calcium is not available in muscle to initiate contraction. Although the precise site or mechanism of action is still controversial,[3] it is clear that the calcium antagonists do decrease systemic vascular resistance by diminishing calcium availability for smooth muscle contraction. Likewise, calcium dependent myocardial contraction and A-V conduction are both altered by the calcium antagonists, but these to a lesser degree than the smooth muscle contractile processes. The overall hemodynamic response to the primary effects of calcium antagonists is dependent on the factors illustrated in figure 1. Probably the most important aspect is the reflex adrenergic mechanisms which counteract the vasodilation and negative inotropic, dromotropic and chromotropic effects. If these mechanisms are present, less hypotension is expected, but if blocked either by adrenergic blocking drugs (e.g., beta blockers) or if the heart is failing and has exhausted its reserve, then depression will be more severe.

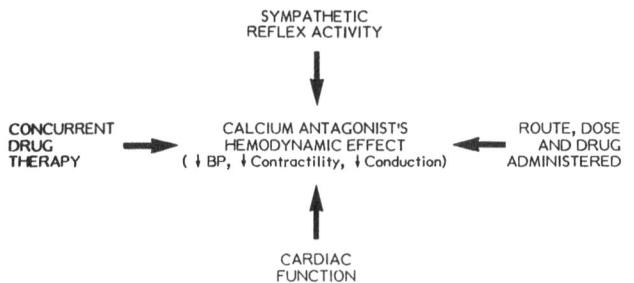

FIGURE 1.

As stated above, the calcium antagonists are a diverse group of compounds, and just as their structures differ so do their respective hemodynamic effects. The relative actions of each are schematically presented in Table II. The differences are even more pronounced when they are given intravenously (as only verapamil can be now, but soon diltiazem and nifedipine will be available for parenteral administration). Note that the primary effect of nifedipine is vasodilation whereas verapamil causes pronounced slowing of A-V conduction. Diltiazem is between these two drugs in most cardiovascular effects. Remember that patients with intact adrenergic reflexes will counteract most of these effects by activation of sympathetic reflex mechanisms (see Fig. 1).

Table II

COMPARISON CARDIOVASCULAR EFFECTS
Ca++ BLOCKERS

	Verapamil	Nifedipine	Diltiazem
Systemic Vasodilation	+	++	+
A-V Conduction Slowing	++	-	+
Negative Inotropism	+	-	-
Heart Rate	±	+	+

Where + = an effect and - = no effect and ± = little or no effect, and ++ = greater effect than +.

Calcium Antagonists and Anesthetic Drugs

There are a large number of potential uses for calcium antagonists in the perioperative period.[1] These include treatment of supraventricular arrhythmias, coronary and cerebral arterial spasm, hypertension, myocardial protection, uterine relaxation, and elective hypotension. Despite the great potential, few of these uses have been reported in man during anesthesia.[12-15] Nevertheless, the interactions of calcium antagonists and various anesthetics have been a relatively active and productive area of laboratory research. Interactions of nifedipine (Table III) and verapamil (Table IV) have been reported with inhalation anesthetics, opiods, and muscle relaxants. There is only one study examining diltiazem.[16]

Table III.

NIFEDIPINE AND DRUG INTERACTIONS

Anesthetic	Interaction	Investigator (Ref #)
Halothane	↓SVR, ↓BP, ↓dP/dt	Tosone (21) Marshall (32) Springman (22) Zaggy (16)
Morphine/N_2O	↓SVR, ↓BP	Springman (22)
Curare	↓twitch	Bikhazi (33)
Pancuronium	↓twitch	Bikhazi (33)
Vecuronium	↓twitch	Bikhazi (33)
Atracurium	↓twitch	Bikhazi (33)

Table IV.

VERAPAMIL AND DRUG INTERACTIONS

Drug	Interaction	Investigator (Reference #)
Halothane	↓BP, ↓SVR, ↑PR ↓dP/dt, ↓CO, ↓BP ↓MAC	Kapur (23) Hantler (25) Norfleet (24) Zaggy (16) Maze (34)
Isoflurane	↓BP, ↓SVR, ↑PR ↓ventricular function	Kapur (26) Kates (14)
Enflurane	↓BP, ↓SVR, ↑PR	Kapur (26)
N_2O	↓BP, ↓dP/dt	Norfleet (24)
Pancuronium	↓muscle twitch	Kraynack (35) Durant (36) Bikhazi (33)
Curare	↓muscle twitch	Bikhazi (33)
Atracurium	↓muscle twitch	Bikhazi (33)
Vecuronium	↓muscle twitch	Bikhazi (33)
Succinylcholine	↓muscle twitch	Durant (36)

54

The interactions of nifedipine with various anesthetics are listed in Table III. The predominant effect has been an "additive type" depression in most hemodynamic parameters, particularly in decreases of SVR and blood pressure. Certainly inhalation anesthetics which interfere with normal calcium dynamics[17-20] would be expected to have an additive effect with calcium antagonists (Fig. 2) and such is the case. These additive effects with inhalation agents are a combination of direct drug effects and inhibition of reflex responses as well (see Fig. 1 for interplay of factors). Tosone showed that if halothane were increased from 1% to 2% that the infusion of 10 mcg/kg of nifedipine produced greater hypotension.[21] This appeared to be because the higher halothane blunted the sympathetic compensatory (tachycardia) response to the decrease in blood pressure. The results of Springman's work revealed that nifedipine (5mcg/kg) produced greater hypotension during halothane (1%) than in morphine-N_2O anesthetized animals.[22] Since morphine does not attenuate compensatory reflexes as halothane dose, the greater nifedipine depression presumably is a result of both the direct depression of halothane and the inhibition of adrenergic reflexes.

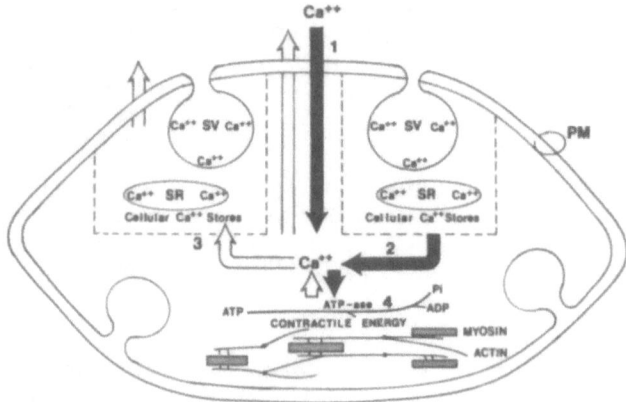

FIGURE 2. Schematic drawing of smooth muscle cell showing calcium flux and possible sites of interference of halothane and nifedipine. Cytoplasmic calcium (Ca^{++}) concentration is increased (black arrows) by entry through the plasma membrane (PM) and released from surface vesicles (SV) or the sarcoplasmic reticulum (SR). When cytoplasmic Ca^{++} concentration is sufficiently high, it activates ATP-ase which splits ATP providing energy for actomyosin interaction and contraction. Cytoplasmic Ca^{++} concentration decreases (white arrows) with return of Ca^{++} to cellular stores and extracellular transport. It is probable that halothane and nifedipine both inhibit Ca^{++} entry (1) and may also interfere with cytoplasmic Ca^{++} flux by reduced SR release (2), storage and reuptake (3), or block ATP-ase and/or the contractile mechanism (4). (Reproduced with permission from the publisher of Anesth Analg and Tosone (reference 21).)

The interaction of verapamil with anesthetics is shown in Table IV. As with nifedipine, additive hemodynamic depression is the usual response. Halothane[16,23-25] as well as enflurane,[14,26] isoflurane[26] and N_2O[24] all tend to add to the decreases in hemodynamic parameters when verapamil is administered. The major difference between interactions of verapamil with inhalation anesthetics and nifedipine with them is that verapamil prolongs the PR interval whereas nifedipine does not. This obviously is important in patients who already have A-V conduction delay, e.g. patients on digoxin and beta adrenergic blockers or with inherent A-V conduction defects.

Although the mechanism is not yet fully understood, verapamil[27] and perhaps other calcium antagonists can prolong the twitch response. Interaction studies (Tables III and IV) show the potential for all muscle relaxants to interact with both verapamil and nifedipine (presumably also diltiazem). Therefore, it is possible that the duration of action of muscle relaxants could be prolonged in patients maintained or given calcium antagonists.

The final point to address is whether or not calcium antagonists should be continued up to operation in patients chronically maintained on them. It has been shown that withdrawal of nifedipine can cause "rebound" coronary artery spasm.[28] Therefore, it appears that discontinuation of therapy is unwarranted unless the potential risks of continuing the therapy (interaction with anesthesia) outweigh the benefits. In a study of 14 patients having coronary bypass surgery, Freis and Lappas[29] reported that nifedipine and propranolol treated patients (n = 7) had significantly greater hypotension and decreased SVR during induction with fentanyl (50 mcg/kg) than untreated patients (n = 7). The decreases in blood pressure and SVR responded to phenylephrine and volume infusion. The FDA permitted Pfizer to put a warning in the Physicians' Desk Reference and package insert of nifedipine which stated:[30]

> Although in most patients, the hypotensive effect of PROCARDIA is modest and well tolerated, occasional patients have had excessive and poorly tolerated hypotension. These responses have usually occurred during initial titration or at the time of subsequent upward dosage adjustment, and may be more likely in patients on concomitant beta blockers.
> Severe hypotension and/or increased fluid volume requirements have been reported in patients receiving PROCARDIA together with a beta blocking agent who underwent coronary artery bypass surgery using high dose fentanyl anesthesia. The interaction with high dose fentanyl appears to be due to the combination of PROCARDIA and a beta blocker, but the possibility that it may occur with PROCARDIA alone, with low doses of fentanyl, in other surgical procedures, or

with other narcotic analgesics cannot be ruled out. In PROCARDIA treated patients where surgery using high dose fentanyl anesthesia is contemplated, the physician should be aware of these potential problems and, if the patient's condition permits, sufficient time (at least 36 hours) should be allowed for PROCARDIA to be washed out of the body prior to surgery.

In an attempt to discover how often, when, and with what anesthetics "severe hypotension" occurred, a questionnaire was submitted to attendees of the Society of Cardiovascular Anesthesiologists Annual Meeting in 1983. Results of the questionnaire are in Table V and reveal that excessive hypotension is rare, occurs at any time during operation and with any anesthetic technique. Furthermore, our data collected prospectively[31] showed that there is no association of blood nifedipine levels with the changes in blood pressure we encountered in anesthetizing 10 CABG patients with diazepam (0.3-0.5 mg/kg) and enflurane (0.5-1.5%). In view of the potential risks of rebound angina and the low incidence of treatable hypotension during anesthesia, it seems prudent to continue patients on calcium antagonists prior to operation.

Table V.

SURVEY RESULTS
1983 MEETING OF SOCIETY OF CARDIOVASCULAR ANESTHESIOLOGISTS

(Number of Respondents = 107)

Number who have seen "severe hypotension" in practice: 30 yes/77 no (31%)

Anesthetic technique used during "severe hypotension":

1	mainly volatile anesthetics
13	high dose fentanyl
16	balanced (modest dose fentanyl, volatile)

When "severe hypotension" occurs:*

15	induction
9	prep
6	prior to CPB
8	during CPB
20	after CPB

Number recommending discontinuation of calcium antagonists more than 24hours before surgery: 9 yes/98 no (8%)

*The occurrence of excessive hypotension occurred at more than one time; therefore, 58 occurrences are reported by the 30 positive respondents.

Conclusion

In summary, nifedipine verapamil, and diltiazem are among the class of drugs called calcium antagonists, but each has a unique spectrum of cardiovascular action. They are very useful compounds and widely prescribed, but their uses during anesthesia are still largely unknown. The concomitant use of calcium antagonists with anesthetics may produce additive hemodynamic depression both because of direct interaction and because anesthetics may blunt the adrenergic reflex responses. When used together, the dose of calcium antagonists and anesthetics should be chosen carefully realizing the potential for drug interaction. There appears to be insufficient data to support the discontinuation of calcium antagonists prior to anesthesia.

References

1. Reves JG, Kissin I, Lell WA, Tosone S: Calcium entry blockers: Uses and implications for the anesthesiologists. Anesthesiology 57:504-518, 1982
2. McAuley BJ, Schroeder JS: The use of diltiazem hydrochloride in cardiovascular disorders. Pharmacotherapy 2:121-133, 1982
3. Braunwald E: Mechanism of action of calcium-channel-blocking agents. N Engl J Med 307:1618-1627, 1982
4. Movsesian MA: Calcium physiology in smooth muscle. Prog Cardiovasc Dis 25:211-224, 1982
5. White BC, Winegar CD, Wilson RF, Hoehner PJ, Trombley JH Jr: Possible role of calcium blockers in cerebral resuscitation: A review of the literature and synthesis for future studies. Crit Care Med 11:202-207, 1983
6. Weiss GB: New Perspectives on Calcium Antagonists. Bethesda, American Physiological Society, 1981
7. McAllister RG Jr: Clinical pharmacokinetics of calcium channel antagonists. J Cardiovasc Pharmacol 4:S340-S345, 1982
8. Covinsky JO, Hamburger SC: Slow channel blockers. South Med J 76:55-64, 1983
9. Fleckenstein A: History of calcium antagonists. Circ Res 52(Part II):I-3-I-17, 1983
10. Triggle DJ, Swamy VC: Calcium antagonists: Some chemical-pharmacologic aspects. Circ Res 52(Part II):I-17-I-28, 1983
11. Klein W, Brandt D, Vrecko K, Harringer M: Role of calcium antagonists in the treatment of essential hypertension. Circ Res 52(Part II):I-174-I-181, 1983
12. Braunwald E: Introduction: Calcium channel blockers. Am J Cardiol 46:1045-1046, 1980
13. Zimpfer M, Fitzal S, Tonczar L: Verapamil as a hypotensive agent during neuroleptanaesthesia. Br J Anaesth 53:885-889, 1981
14. Kates RA, Kaplan JA, McKeown PP, Freniere S: The cardiovascular effects of verapamil administration during coronary artery bypass graft surgery. Anesthesiology 57:A1, 1982
15. Kopman EA: Intravenous verapamil to relieve pulmonary congestion in patients with mitral valve disease. Anesthesiology 58:374-376, 1983
16. Zaggy AP, Kates RA, Norfleet EA, Mueller RA, Heath KR: The comparative cardiovascular effects of verapamil, nifedipine, and diltiazem during halothane anesthesia. SCA Fifth Annual Meeting, San Diego, CA, April 1983, pp 95-96

17. Komai H, Rusy BF: Effect of halothane on rested-state and potentiated-state contractions in rabbit papillary muscle: Relationship to negative inotropic action. Anesth Analg 61:403-409, 1982

18. Blanck TJ, Thompson M: Calcium transport by cardiac sarcoplasmic reticulum: Modulation of halothane action by substrate concentration and pH. Anesth Analg 60:390-394, 1981

19. Lynch C, Vogel S, Sperelakis N: Halothane depresses cardiac slow action potentials. Anesthesiology 49:407-413, 1978

20. Altura BM, Altura BT, Carella A, et al: Vascular smooth muscle and general anesthetics. Fed Proc 39:1584-1591, 1980

21. Tosone SR, Reves JG, Kissin I, Smith LR, Fournier SE: Hemodynamic responses to nifedipine in halothane anesthetized dogs. Anesth Analg 62: 000-000, 1983 (in press)

22. Springman SR, Redon D, Rusy BF: The effect of nifedipine on the circulation during morphine N_2O and halothane anesthesia in dogs. Anesth Analg 62:284-285, 1983

23. Kapur PA, Flacke WE: Epinephrine-induced arrhythmias and cardiovascular function after verapamil during halothane anesthesia in the dog. Anesthesiology 55:218-225, 1981

24. Norfleet EA, Heath KR, Kopp VJ, Sprague DH, Corke BC: Verapamil - different cardiovascular responses during N_2O analgesia and halothane anesthesia. Anesthesiology 57:A75, 1982

25. Hantler CB, Clifford BD, Kroll DA, Knight PR: Verapamil does have prolonged interactions with halothane. Anesthesiology 57:A2, 1982

26. Kapur PA, Flacke WE: Lack of correlation of verapamil plasma level with cumulative protective effects against halothane - epinephrine ventricular arrhythmias. J Cardiovasc Pharmacol 4:652-657, 1982

27. Lawson NW, Kraynack BJ, Gintautas J: Neuromuscular and electrocardiographic responses to verapamil in dogs. Anesth Analg 62:50-54, 1983

28. Schick EC Jr, Liang C, Heupler FA Jr, et al: Randomized withdrawal from nifedipine: Placebo-controlled study in patients with coronary artery spasm. Am Heart J 104:690-697, 1982

29. Freis ES, Lappas DG: Chronic administration of calcium entry blockers and the cardiovascular responses to high doses of fentanyl in man. Anesthesiology 57:A295, 1982

30. Physicians' Desk Reference, 37th Edition. Oradell, Medical Economics Company Inc., 1983, p 1580

31. Reves JG, Barker S, Smith LR: Significance of nifedipine plasma levels and hemodynamic changes during anesthesia induction. (Abstract) Anesthesiology (in press)

32. Marshall AG, Kissin I, Reves JG, Bradley EL Jr, Blackstone EH: Interaction between negative inotropic effects of halothane and nifedipine in the isolated rat heart. J Cardiovasc Pharmacol (in press)

33. Bikhazi GB, Leung I, Foldes FF: Interaction of neuromuscular blocking agents with calcium channel blockers. Anesthesiology 57:A268, 1982

34. Maze M, Mason DM: Verapamil decreases the MAC for halothane in dogs. Anesth Analg 62:274, 1983

35. Kraynack BJ, Lawson NW, Gintautas J: Verapamil reduces indirect muscle twitch amplitude and potentiates pancuronium in vitro. Anesthesiology 57:A265, 1982

36. Durant NN, Nguyen N, Briscoe JR, Katz RL: Potentiation of pancuronium and succinylcholine by verapamil. Anesthesiology 57:A267, 1982

RATIONALE AND PROBLEMS OF PULMONARY VASCULAR PRESSURE MONITORING: AN UPDATE

NATHAN L. PACE, M.D.

Drs. Swan and Ganz added their names to popular medical culture by creating and publicizing a practical, bedside pulmonary artery (PA) catheter in 1970.[1] Since then, anesthesiologists and other acute care physicians have become proficient in "Swanning" their patients.   An accumulation of review articles have provided details in the use of pulmonary artery catheters.[2-8] There is a continual expansion of new patient groups in which pulmonary vascular monitoring is used.   Recent reviews address the use of Swan-Ganz catheters in critically ill obstetric and pediatric patients.[9-10] Several reports now summarize the expected complications associated with pulmonary vascular monitoring.[11-14] Fortunately, catheter complications are generally transient and without long term morbidity.   Nevertheless, case reports of bizarre complications continue to appear.[15]

Familiarity with the pulmonary artery catheter enables physicians to generate enormous quantities of numbers including: repetitive measurement of pulmonary arterial pressures, cardiac output, and mixed venous oxygen saturation.   Some of the limitations of accuracy and of interpretation of catheter measurements are not well understood and will be discussed in this review.

The raison d'etre of PA catheters is to measure the "wedge" pressure. Pulmonary wedge pressure refers to the pressure measured when a catheter is impacted in a branch of the PA and free communication is still present between the catheter tip and the capillary-venous compartment of the lung. The motionless blood between the catheter tip and left atrium serves as a fluid filled manometer communicating left heart pressures to a right heart catheter. The balloon of a Swan-Ganz PA catheter may be intermittently inflated to "float" the catheter tip into the wedge position. The wedge pressure is referred to as the pulmonary artery occlusion pressure (PAOP) in this review. PAOP is often equated with left sided filling pressures.

The pressure waveforms of pulmonary artery catheters are viewed after electronic transduction and monitor display. The faithfulness of transmission of the waveform will depend on the fidelity of the cannula, the connecting tubing, and the transducer system.[16],[17] The measurement of pulmonary arterial pressures is more difficult in the presence of the large pressure fluctuations associated with breathing. Some have recommended the use of paper graphic output to measure pressures rather than electronic sampling.[18] Normal fluctuations in pulmonary arterial pressures occur over time; i.e. the wedge pressure might vary as much as 4 mm Hg in critically ill patients during periods of apparent hemodynamic stability.[19]

Artifactual PAOP readings can be produced by an over inflated balloon occluding the catheter tip and is easily recognized as an "overwedge" pattern. Partial wedging of the catheter tip is difficult to detect; it probably occurs when an eccentric balloon inflation does not totally occlude the vessel lumen or when the balloon is straddling a vessel bifurcation. Artifactual PAOP's are higher than the true PAOP. Recent work by Morris et al suggests that artifactual, partially wedged PAOP's are frequent in critically ill patients.[20] When there is a question of validity in PAOP measurement, three criteria of true wedge tracing must be met: First, a change in the phasic contour of the pulmonary artery waveform should occur with wedging. Second, there should be a fall in mean pressure with wedging. Third, the PO_2 of blood withdrawn from the wedged PA catheter should be higher than a simultaneous arterial PO_2. [The ability to withdraw blood from the pulmonary capillaries via a wedged catheter may in the future have some utility in the investigation and diagnosis of the adult respiratory distress syndrome.[21]]

By convention, PAOP should be read at the end of expiration. In the anesthetized patient it is almost always possible to create apnea of sufficient duration to get a stable PAOP. By contrast, the spontaneously breathing patient may have wide shifts in intrathoracic pressure which can be partially transmitted to the pulmonary artery. It may be impossible to pick the end expiratory moment of the PAOP trace. Since the change in PAOP observed over the respiratory cycle may be 20-40 mm Hg, the importance of choosing the proper end expiratory point is obvious.[22] One solution is to record simultaneously PAOP and airway pressure and use the end expiratory point of the airway pressure trace to choose the end expiratory PAOP.[23] An airway thermistor has been developed which detects end expiration and allows automated measurement of PAOP.[24]

The actual filling pressure of a cardiac chamber is the transmural distending pressure which is defined as the inside pressure minus the outside pressure. The inside pressure might be the central venous pressure (CVP) or the PAOP. The outside pressure is the pericardial pressure. This pericardial pressure is similiar to but not identical with intrapleural pressure and is slightly below atmospheric pressure in the quietly breathing patient; thus CVP and PAOP referenced to atmosphere are reasonably accurate. When a patient is being treated with PEEP, variable amounts of airway pressure may be transmitted through the lung parenchyma, thus raising intrapleural and pericardial pressure. Under these conditions, PAOP and CVP referenced to atmospheric pressure will overestimate transmural pressure.[25] Attempts to directly or indirectly measure intrapleural pressure are fraught with technical problems. Measurement of PAOP and CVP during a brief period of PEEP removal will reflect a hemodynamic state other than the one of interest. Also, without a prudent protocol for an increased FiO_2 during PEEP removal, some patients are likely to become hypoxemic during PAOP measurements.[26] At present there is no practical method of measuring transmural pressures during PEEP.[27]

Another adverse effect of PEEP involves the alveolar waterfall phenomenon. In regions of lung in which alveolar pressure is higher than pulmonary venous pressure, but less than pulmonary artery pressure, the alveolar vessels partially collapse and blood flow becomes independant of the more negative downstream pulmonary venous pressure.[28] Under the no flow conditions of a catheter wedged into the artery of such a lung region, the catheter tip pressure will fall to the level of the pressure of the collapsible alveolar segment and not to the more negative downstream pulmonary venous pressure. This is called an alveolar waterfall phenomenon. The presence or absence of a PAOP to pulmonary venous pressure discrepancy will depend on the complex relationship of: 1) the height of the PA catheter tip above the left atrium during wedging, 2) the left atrial pressure (LAP), and 3) the level of PEEP. Unfortunately the presence or absence of a PAOP to LAP discrepancy is not discernable with only a PA catheter. Recent experimental work does give some confidence that PAOP remains an accurate reflection of LAP during spontaneous breathing with PEEP up to 20 mmHg.[29] A partial protection of PAOP estimates of LAP is also noted during mechanical ventilation with PEEP of non compliant lungs.[29] A recent clinical study confirmed the PAOP to LAP discrepancy during mechanical ventilation in patients with compliant lungs.[30] In 43% of 30 post operative open heart surgery patients, the tip of the pulmonary artery catheter was at or above the left atrium with the patient in the supine positon; with increasing PEEP, there was an increasing difference between PAOP and LAP.[30]

We are interested in PAOP's for two reasons. First, the PAOP gives an estimate of pulmonary venous pressure which is one of the determinants of transcapillary water flux as described by the Starling equation. Second, the PAOP hopefully will describe left ventricular filling. In normal patients, PAOP, LAP and Left Ventricular End Diastolic Pressure (LVEDP) are essentially interchangeable. It is now apparent that there are clinical circumstances during which PAOP does not accurately reflect LAP or LVEDP. For about the first 16 hours following open heart surgery, PAOP systematically overestimates LAP by 5 to 8 mm Hg.[31] There is no explanation yet for this observation.[31]

Following myocardial infarction, atrial contraction makes a greater contribution to left ventricular filling; the atrial kick at end diastole raises left ventricular pressure much higher than LAP (LVEDP $\geq$ LAP + 10 mm Hg). PAOP now reflects the left ventricular diastolic pressure prior to atrial contraction and is a poor estimate of left ventricular end diastolic pressure, but still provides reliable information about the potential for pulmonary edema. The lower the cardiac output, the more important is atrial contraction for ventricular filling and the less reliable is mean PAOP for estimating LVEDP. In conditions known to produce a PAOP to LVEDP discrepancy, the use of left ventricular stroke work calculations should be considered critically.

One can usually see and measure left atrial phasic variations in the wedge trace called the a, c, and v waves. The most important of these is the v wave. The presence of large v waves is commonly interpreted as diagnostic of significant mitral regurgitation.[32,33] More systematic study has confirmed that mitral regurgitation is the most common cause of large v waves; unfortunately, large v̇ waves are neither highly sensitive or specific for severe mitral regurgitation.[34,35]

Even if PAOP perfectly reflects LVEDP, a further reservation must be made about interpretation of PAOP's. It is widely accepted that the Frank-Starling law applies to the intact human heart; i.e., at any given functional state, the force of ventricular contraction is dependent upon its end - diastolic volume or end- diastolic wall tension. For want of a technique for routine ventricular volume determination, investigators and clincans have relied on LVEDP as an index of left ventricular end diastolic volume and wall tension.

During diastole, cardiac relaxation (an energy dependent process) occurs. The left ventricle then fills passively and the pressure developed is exponentially related to the volume. An elevated LVEDP is commonly taken to signify the presence of increased left ventricular volume and thus left ventricular failure. A normal LVEDP is assumed to be evidence against the presence of left ventricular failure. In fact, apparent left ventricular function as reflected by LVEDP can change in many ways. Among them are a true change in the left ventricular contractile state or a change in the diastolic properties of the left ventricle.[36] For example, following acute myocardial infarction impaired ventricular relaxation and decreased diastolic ventricular compliance may account in part for an elevation in LVEDP without any change in ventricular volume. Also, it is probable that high levels of PEEP may cause right ventricular dilation, shift the interventricular septum toward the left ventricle, lower left ventricular compliance, and raise LVEDP with an actual reduction in left ventricular diastolic volume. This failure of changes in PAOP to properly estimate changes in left ventricular end diastolic volume has now been shown in patients with acute myocardial infarction and sepsis[37] and following myocardial revascularizaiton.[38] Under these conditions it may be incorrect to assume that an elevated LVEDP represents an impairment of myocardial contractility. Unfortunately, we have no practical way of determining changes in ventricular diastolic properties.

I have detailed some of the circumstances in which PAOP is not a true reflection of left ventricular filling and function or pulmonary venous pressure. PAOP measurements must be used with caution. Other indices of circulatory adequacy (arterial pressure, CVP, PvO_2, organ function, etc.) will help resolve some of the uncertainty. Routine intraoperative use of echocardiographic or radionuclide ventriculography may in the future be possible, allowing frequent measurement of ventricular end diastolic volumes,thus avoiding tenuous estimations of heart filling by PAOP measurement.

REFERENCES

1. Swan HJC, Ganz W, Forrester J, Marcus H, Diamond G, Chonette D: Catheterization of the heart in man with the use of a flow-directed balloon-tipped catheter. N Engl J Med 1970;283:447-451.
2. Swan HJC, Ganz W: Use of balloon flotation catheters in critically ill patients. Surg Clin N Am 1975;55:501-520.
3. Buchbinder N, Ganz W: Hemodynamic monitoring: Invasive techniques. Anesthesiology 1976;45:146-155.
4. Gorlin R: Current concepts in cardiology: Practical cardiac hemo- dynamics. N Engl J Med 1977;296:203-205.
5. Lappas DG, Powell WM Jr, Daggett WM: Cardiac dysfunction in the perioperative period. Pathophysiology, diagnosis, and treatment. Anesthesiology 1977;47:117-137.
6. Pace NL: A critique of flow-directed pulmonary arterial catheter- ization. Anesthesiology 1977;47:455-465.
7. Swan HJC, Ganz W: Measurement of right atrial and pulmonary arterial pressures and cardiac output: Clinical application of hemodynamic monitoring. Adv Intern Med 1982;27:453-473.
8. Moser KM, Spragg RG: Use of the balloon-tipped pulmonary artery catheter in pulmonary disease. Ann Intern Med 1983;98:53-58.
9. Cotton DB, Benedetti TJ: Use of the Swan-Ganz catheter in obstetrics and gynecology. Obstet Gynecol 1980;56:641-645.
10. Weesner KM, Rocchini AP, Rosenthal A: Use of balloon-tipped cath- eters in the critically ill child. Clin Pediatr (Phil) 1982; 21:146-149.
11. Elliot GC, Zimmerman GA, Clemmer TP: Complications of pulmonary artery catheterization in the care of critically ill patients. Chest 1979; 76:647-652.
12. Puri VK, Carlson RW, Bander JJ, Weil MH: Complications of vascular catheterization in the critically ill: A prospective study. Crit Care Med 1980;8:495-499.
13. Quinn K, Quebbeman EJ: Pulmonary artery pressure monitoring in the surgical intensive care unit: Benefits vs difficulties: Arch Surg 1981;116:872-876.
14. Davies MJ, Cronin KD, Domaingue CM: Pulmonary artery catheteriza- tion. An assessment of risks and benefits in 220 surgical patients. Anaesth Intensive Care 1982;10:9-14.
15. Smith GB, Willatts SM: A hazard of Swan-Ganz catheterization. Anaesthesia 1981;36:398-401.

16. Gardner RM: Direct blood pressure measurements - dynamic response requirements. Anesthesiology 1981;54:227-236.
17. Runciman WB, Rutten AJ, Ilsley AH: An evaluation of blood pressure measurement. Anaesth Intensive Care 1981;9:314-325.
18. Maran AG: Variables in pulmonary capillary wedge pressure: variation with intrathoracic pressure, graphic and digital recorders. Crit Care Med 1980;8:102-105.
19. Nemens EJ, Woods SL: Normal fluctuations in pulmonary artery and pulmonary capillary wedge pressures in acutely ill patients. Heart Lung 1982;11:393-398.
20. Morris AH, Hol R: Pulmonary wedge pressure - A difficult measurement. Am Rev Respir Dis 1980;121:170.
21. Allen WG, Olsen GN, Williams WH, Yergin BM: Recovery of embolized albumin microspheres from the pulmonary microvasculature using a wedged balloon-tipped catheter. Crit Care Med 1983;11:261264.
22. Teeple E, Ghia JN: An elevated pulmonary wedge pressure resulting from an upper respiratory obstruction in an obese patient. Anesthesiology 1983;59:66-68.
23. Berryhill RE, Benumof JL, Rauscher LA: Pulmonary vascular pressure reading at the end of exhalation. Anesthesiology 1978;49:365-368.
24. Oden R, Mitchell MM, Benumof JL: Detection of end-exhalation period by airway thermistor: an approach to automated pulmonary artery pressure measurement. Anesthesiology 1983;58:467-471.
25. Qvist J, Pontoppidan H, Wilson RS, Lowenstein E, Laver MB. Hemodynamic responses to mechanical ventilation with PEEP: The effect of hypervolemia. Anesthesiology 1975;42:45-55.
26. de Campo T, Civetta JM: The effect of short-term discontinuation of high-level PEEP in patients with acute respiratory failure. Crit Care Med 1979;7:47-49.
27. Geer RT. Interpretation of pulmonary-artery wedge pressure when PEEP is used. Anesthesiology 1977;46:383-384.
28. Roy R, Powers SR, Feustel PJ, Dutton RE. Pulmonary wedge catheterization during positive end-expiratory pressure ventilation in the dog. Anesthesiology 1977;46:385-390.
29. Berryhill RE, Benumof JL. PEEP - induced discrepancy between pulmonary arterial wedge pressure and left arterial pressure: The effects of controlled vs spontaneous ventilation and compliant vs noncompliant lungs in the dog. Anesthesiology 1979;51:303-308.
30. Shasby DM, Dauber IM, Pfister S, Anderson JT, Carson SB, Manart F, Hyers TM: Swan-Ganz catheter location and left atrial pressure determine the accuracy of the wedge pressure when positive end-expiratory pressure is used. Chest 1981;80:666-670.
31. Mammana RB, Hiro S, Levitsky S, Thomas PA, Plachetka J: Inaccuracy of pulmonary capillary wedge pressure when compared to left atrial pressure in the early postsurgical period. J Thorac Cardiovasc Surg 1982;84:420-425.
32. Meister SG, Helfant RH: Rapid bedside differentiation of ruptured interventricular septum from acute mitral insufficiency. N Engl J Med 1972;287:1024-1025.
33. Forrester JS, Diamond G, Freedman S, Allen HN, Parmley WW, Matloff J, Swan HJ. Silent mitral insufficiency in acute myocardial infarction. Circulation 1971;44:877-883.
34. Fuchs RM, Heuser RR, Yin FCP, Brinker JA. Limitation of pulmonary wedge v waves in diagnosing mitral regurgitation. Am J Cardiol 1982;49:849-854.

35. Pichard AD, Kay R, Smith H, Rentrop P, Holt J, Gorlin R. Large v waves in the pulmonary wedge pressure tracing in the absence of mitral regurgitation. Am J Cardiol 1982;50:1044-1050.
36. Lewis BS, Gotsman MS. Current concepts of left ventricular relaxation and compliance. Am Heart J 1980;99:101-112.
37. Calvin E, Driedger AA, Sibbald WJ: Does the pulmonary capillary wedge pressure predict left ventricular preload in critically ill patients? Crit Care Med 1981;9:437-443.
38. Ellis RJ, Mangano DT, VanDyke DC: Relationship of wedge pressure to end-diastolic volume in patients undergoing myocardial revascularization. J Thorac Cardiovasc Surg 1979;78:605-613.

HIGH DOSE OPIOIDS FOR CORONARY ARTERY SURGERY

NORBERT P. DE BRUIJN M.D., SIMON DE LANGE M.B.B.S., FFARCS, Ph.D.

The popularity of the narcotic analgesics in coronary artery surgery is mainly based on their ability to provide "stress-free" anesthesia and on their alleged minimal cardiac effects.
Lowenstein et al (1) reported the first series of patients anesthetized for aortic valve replacement with high dose morphine. They observed increases in cardiac index, stroke index, central venous pressure and pulmonary arterial pressure as well as a significant decrease in peripheral vascular resistance and they concluded that large doses of morphine may be used with safety in patients with minimal circulatory reserve.
There have been a host of experiments done in isolated hearts, studying the effects of morphine and the synthetic opioids (2, 3, 4, 5) and in all of these studies it was found that the opioids caused a dose related depression of cardiac performance. In all these experiments however prodigious doses of narcotics were used which makes comparison with studies in intact animals or humans difficult or even impossible.
When the high dose morphine technique had been used for a while it appeared that there were a number of problems related to its use mainly in patients with good cardiovascular reserve. Of these problems the high incidence of hypertension and hypotension were the most important ones.
The above features of high dose morphine limited its use and favoured the introduction of high-dose fentanyl anesthesia for coronary artery surgery. Lunn et al (6) described the hemodynamic effects of fentanyl 25-75 ug.kg^{-1}. They reported small decreases in pulmonary artery pressure, pulmonary capillary pressure and in systemic and pulmonary vascular resistance. There was no significant change in heart rate, cardiac output or right atrial pressure at any time.
Fentanyl also appeared to result in less prolonged respiratory depression than morphine (7). Stanley et al (8) used an average of 71 ug.kg^{-1} of fentanyl in patients undergoing coronary artery bypass grafting, which was observed to produce small but significant reductions in heart rate and mean systemic arterial pressure, but stroke volume, cardiac output and pulmonary vascular resistance were unchanged. In short the advantages of high dose fentanyl appeared to include greater hemodynamic stability, no evidence of histamine release and shorter post-operative respiratory depression. Also high dose fentanyl techniques have been shown to inhibit the cortisol response throughout

surgery, whereas plasma levels of ADH and GH where still elevated during CPB and during surgery after CPB.

After the initial enthusiasm for high dose fentanyl techniques untoward reports about this method began to appear. Chest wall rigidity not uncommonly precedes loss of consciousness at induction with fentanyl (9, 10). Our impression is that the rate of administration of the opioid may be important to minimize this rigidity. Precurarisation does not reduce the incidence of the rigidity but may result in less severe rigidity.

The high dose fentanyl techniques provide a very stable induction but hemodynamic reaction requiring supplemental anesthesia is frequently reported at the time of skin incision, sternal split, aortic root dissection and after weaning of cardiopulmonary bypass. Various techniques have been tried to cope with this problem, including progressively higher doses of fentanyl (up to 160 ug.kg^{-1}). Nitrous oxide is usually avoided because it causes myocardial depression in combination with opioids and because it exacerbates air embolism. Supplementary agents used include intravenous anesthetics (thiopental, etomidate, diazepam, lorazepam), volatile anesthetics (halothane, enflurane, isoflurane) or vasodilators (nitroprusside, nitroglycerin, regitine). Although very high doses of fentanyl may decrease the incidence of intra-operative hypertensive responses (11), this approach may lead to an undesirable increase in the duration of post-operative sedation and respiratory depression.

Recently attempts have been made to alleviate a number of the intra-operative problems discussed above, by means of a continuous infusion of fentanyl (12). It appears that this technique will enable us to attain stable anesthetic levels at a predictable fentanyl plasma level. Studies of the dose-response relationship will be facilitated by this technique.

Little has been published about the post-operative effects of high-dose fentanyl for coronary artery surgery. In our experience these patients frequently appear to become agitated and disoriented in the ICU. Also a recurrence of muscle rigidity is seen not infrequently in our post-operative cardiac patients.

Sonntag et al (13) reported that four out of nine patients showed signs of awareness during coronary artery surgery when anesthetized with an average of 127 ug.kg^{-1} fentanyl for the entire operation. They also observed myocardial lactate production in five of their patients. These data indicate that high doses of fentanyl by itself are not able to produce optimal anesthesia and optimal cardiovascular dynamics. There are however a number critisms possible with regards to this study. In our experience 10 mg diazepam orally which the authors used for premedication is an inadequate dose. Also the authors claim to have continued beta-receptor antagonists (pindolol) but in our opinion administration of pindolol at 10:00 p.m. the night prior to surgery as they did, will not provide adequate beta-blockade at the time of surgery. Finally it is difficult to draw conclusions from measurements of myocardial lactate because these measurements only provide a very global indication about the status of the myocardium, while especially in patients with coronary artery disease, regional differences may be of much greater importance. Still this study again emphasizes that there are a number of problems with the high dose fentanyl technique.

In view of the problems with high dose fentanyl, a number of new congeners of fentanyl have been studied recently. Alfentanil and sufentanil afforded a rapid induction of anesthesia in cardiac and general surgical patients, with excellent hemodynamic stability and allowing stress-free intubation (14, 15, 16).

Alfentanil, used as a sole anesthetic agent during coronary artery surgery resulted in a rapid induction and rapid recovery from anesthesia. Administered intermittantly as intravenous bolus doses, it does not seem to confer any increased hemodynamic stability compared to fentanyl. Continuous infusion of alfentanil was shown to be superior to frequent boluses of the drug in preventing hypertension and minimizing the need for antihypertensive supplements (15). de Lange et al (16) showed that both sufentanil and alfentanil as sole anesthetic agents result in stable cardiovascular dynamics, block increases in plasma cortisol throughout the operation and prevent increases in plasma catecholamine levels up to, but not during and after cardiopulmonary bypass in patients undergoing coronary artery surgery. These drugs were also capable of blocking rises in ADH and GH levels throughout surgery (17).

Sebel et al (18) studied the effects of 15 $ug.kg^{-1}$ sufentanil on cardiovascular dynamics in humans and observed decreases in systolic and mean systemic arterial bloodpressure as well as a decrease in systemic vascular resistance. Systemic diastolic arterial pressure increased significantly after sternotomy.

In conclusion in spite of the reported imperfections high dose opioid techniques for coronary artery surgery appear to provide an adequate overall anesthetic management of these patients. New techniques of administration of fentanyl may still improve its performances and the newer opioids alfentanil and sufentanil appear to be quite attractive alternatives although they have not yet been studied as extensively as fentanyl.

References
 1. Lowenstein E, Hallowel P, Levine FH et al
    Cardiovascular reponse to large doses of intravenous morphine in man.
    N. Engl. J. Med. 281: 1389, 1969

 2. Sullivan DL, Wong KC
    The effects of morphine on the isolated heart during normothermia and hypothermia.
    Anesthesiology 38: 550, 1973

3. Goldberg AH, Padget CH
   Comparative effects of morphine and fentanyl on isolated
   heart muscle.
   Anesth. Analg. 48: 978, 1969

4. Strauer BE
   Contractile responses to morphine, piritramide,
   meperidine and fentanyl. A comparative study of effects
   on the isolated ventricular myocardium.
   Anesthesiology 37: 304, 1972

5. Siepmann HJ, Hartun E
   Action of alfentanil and fentanyl on the mechanics of
   isolated papillary muscle.
   7th World Congress of Anesthesiologists, Hamburg,
   September 1980, 290

6. Lunn JK, Stanley TH, Eisele J et al
   High-dose fentanyl anesthesia for coronary artery
   surgery: Plasma fentanyl concentrations and influence of
   nitrous oxide on cardiovascular responses.
   Anesth. Analg. 58: 390, 1979

7. Murphy MR, Olson WA, Hug CC
   Pharmacokinetics of 3H fentanyl in the dog anesthetized
   with enflurane.
   Anesthesiology 50: 13, 1979

8. Stanley TH, Philbin DH, Coggins CH
   Fentanyl-oxygen anesthesia for coronary artery surgery:
   cardiovascular and antidiuretic hormone responses.
   Canad. Anaesth. Soc. J. 26: 168, 1979

9. Comstock MK, Scamman FL, Carter JG et al
   Rigidity and hypercarbia on fentanyl-oxygen induction.
   Anesthesiology 51: S3, 1979

10. Waller JC, Hug CC, Nagle DM et al
    Hemodynamic changes during fentanyl-oxygen anesthesia for
    coronary artery bypass operations.
    Anesthesiology 55: 212, 1981

11. Wynands JE, Townsend GE, Ping Wong et al
    Blood pressure response and plasma fentanyl
    concentrations during high- and very high-dose fentanyl
    anesthesia for coronary artery surgery.
    Anesth. Analg. 62: 661, 1983

12. Moldenhauer CC, Hug CC
    Continuous infusion of fentanyl for cardiac surgery.
    Anesth. Analg. 61: 206, 1982

13. Sonntag H, Larsen R, Hilfiker O et al
    Myocardial blood flow and oxygen consumption during high-
    dose fentanyl anesthesia in patients with coronary artery
    disease.
    Anesthesiology 56: 417, 1982

14. Nauta J, de Lange S, Koopman D et al
    Anesthetic induction with alfentanil: a new short-acting
    narcotic analgesic.
    Anesth. Analg. 61: 267, 1982

15. de Lange S, de Bruijn NP, Stanley TH et al
    Alfentanil-oxygen anesthesia comparison of continuous
    infusion and frequent bolus techniques for coronary
    artery surgery.
    Anesthesiology 55: A42, 1981

16. de Lange S, Stanley TH, Boscoe MJ
    Comparison of sufentanil-oxygen and fentanyl-oxygen for
    coronary artery surgery.
    Anesthesiology 56: 112, 1982

17. de Lange S, Boscoe MJ, Stanley TH et al
    Anti-diuretic and growth-hormone responses during
    coronary artery surgery with sufentanil-oxygen and
    alfentanil-oxygen anesthesia in man.
    Anesth. Analg. 61: 434, 1982

18. Sebel P. Bovill J
    Cardiovascular effects of sufentanil.
    Anesth. Analg. 61: 115, 1981

RATIONAL USE OF INHALATION AGENTS FOR CORONARY ARTERY SURGERY

THEODORE H. STANLEY, M.D.

The recent enthusiasm for high doses of fentanyl as the sole "anesthetic" or major analgesic supplement in patients with cardiac disease has made some clinicians reduce the frequency and concentration of their employment of potent inhalation anesthetics for cardiac surgery.[1-3] In spite of these changes in clinical practice, it is doubtful whether inhalation anesthetics will ever be totally eliminated as supplements or, in some patients, as sole anesthetics for heart operations. The reason for this is simple: Inhalation anesthetics have unique characteristics that are often not only highly desirable, but considering the alternative, sometimes absolutely necessary in patients with a variety of cardiac pathologies but perhaps most importantly in patients with coronary artery disease.

The objectives of this manuscript will be to focus on the rationale of using inhalation anesthesia and potent inhalation anesthetics for cardiac surgical procedures, particularly patients with coronary artery disease undergoing coronary artery bypass grafting (CABG) operations.

A. Myocardial Oxygen Supply-Demand Considerations

More than 15 percent of the adult population in North America (approximately 40 million people) are estimated to have coronary artery disease (CAD) and somewhere between 175,000-200,000 undergo coronary artery bypass operations each year.[4] Since the major physiological problem in patients with CAD is inadequate myocardial oxygen supply for myocardial oxygen demand,[5,6] it's rational to consider anesthetic techniques that either increase oxygen supply or decrease demand during corrective surgery in these patients. Theoretically myocardial oxygen supply could be increased by increasing aortic diastolic pressure (and thus coronary artery blood flow), by using selective coronary artery vasodilators or by increasing oxygen content in blood perfusing the heart.[5,6] Unfortunately, none of these theoretical possibilities is easy to achieve and/or problem free. An increase in aortic diastolic blood pressure may increase coronary artery blood flow but it also increases left ventricular wall tension, a major determinant of myocardial oxygen demand.[6] Selective coronary artery vasodilators are frequently not selective enough and thus can result in decreases in aortic blood pressure (and coronary artery blood flow) and/or are often already being used to maximum effect preoperatively. In most patients coronary artery oxygen content can only be improved by increasing the amount of oxygen dissolved in blood (increasing PaO_2). Although increases in PaO_2 are easily achievable via increases in F_IO_2, the maximum increase in content possible at atmosphere pressure is somewhat less than 2 ml/100 ml of blood (0.3 ml/100 torr O_2 x 600 torr) or approximately 20% (20 ml to 22 ml/100 ml blood). Because of problems with prolonged high inspired concentrations of oxygen and all of these difficulties of increasing oxygen supply to the myocardium, most clinicians usually concentrate on reducing myocardial oxygen demand rather than increasing myocardial oxygen supply during anesthesia.

The major determinants of myocardial oxygen demand (consumption) are external myocardial work (ventricular pressure x flow), myocardial contractility and heart rate.[5,6] A recent study has shown that inhalation anesthetic (halothane) induced myocardial depression decreases myocardial ischemia secondary to experimental coronary artery occlusion.[8] Since all inhalation agents depress ventricular pressure, cardiac output and myocardial contractility and some also depress heart rate[9-13] and myocardial oxygen consumption,[8,14-20] numerous investigators and clinicians have suggested that inhalation anesthetic induced myocardial depression is desirable in patients with coronary artery disease.[7,8,14-16] There are, of course, the risks of myocardial depression. Chief among these risks is hypotension significant enough to decrease coronary artery blood flow. Because stenotic segments of coronary arteries cannot dilate in response to decreases in coronary perfusion pressure, flow to tissue distal to these stenotic segments is more pressure dependent than tissue in normal coronary arteries.[15] Thus only moderate decreases in arterial blood pressure are desirable if perfusion to subendocardial tissues (the tissues usually most at risk to ischemia) is to be maintained. Of course an important question is, what is a moderate decrease in arterial blood pressure? The obvious answer is a decrease in pressure that decreases external heart work and oxygen demand but does not decrease coronary artery blood flow. Unfortunately, the advantages (if any) and degree of moderate hypotension that is optimal probably varies significantly from patient to patient depending on preoperative hemodynamics, degree of coronary artery disease and a host of other factors which are difficult to evaluate. Therefore it is imperative that careful monitoring for signs of ischemia be initiated before induction of anesthesia and maintained throughout the anesthetic and early postoperative periods.

Although few well controlled studies evaluating halothane, enflurane and isoflurane as elective myocardial depressants in patients with CAD have been performed, there are data available indicating that these agents produce hypotension by different mechanisms. Delaney and co-workers have demonstrated that the primary action of enflurane is to reduce systemic vascular resistance.[17,18] In contrast, halothane appears to have little effect on systemic vascular resistance and acts primarily as a depressant of myocardial contractility. Other data indicate that isoflurane produces hypotension in a manner more similar to enflurane than halothane.[13,17,18]

One of the risks of moderate hypotension is reflex tachycardia. Approximately 85% of total coronary artery blood flow occurs during diastole and almost 100 % of subendocardial blood flow occurs during this period. Increases in heart rate shorten diastole and therefore decrease time for coronary artery perfusion. Decreases in heart rate do the opposite and consequently are desirable in patients with CAD. Tachycardia not only decreases coronary artery perfusion but also increases myocardial oxygen demand. Thus avoiding tachycardia and promoting bradycardia are of profound importance during anesthesia in patients with CAD undergoing open-heart operations. There are data which indicate that reflex tachycardia occurs more frequently during isoflurane than halothane or enflurane.[18] The exact mechanism producing these changes in heart rate is not clearly defined. However, recent clinical experience indicates tachycardia with isoflurane can often, though not always, be easily prevented or treated with small increments (100 ug) of fentanyl intravenously.

Halothane, in contrast to either isoflurane or enflurane, decreases heart rate.[11,17] Although this may be considered an advantage when comparing the agents for patients with CAD undergoing open heart surgery, the magnitude (usually minimal) and significance of this bradycardia on the overall decrease in myocardial oxygen consumption must be balanced against the "other effects" of halothane. The influence of these "other effects", including a higher likelihood of significant ventricular arrhythmias and more severe depression of myocardial contractility and cardiac output, on coronary artery perfusion is an important consideration in choosing which potent inhalation agent will be used.[18,19]

In a comparative study evaluating enflurane and halothane in patients with CAD undergoing coronary artery bypass grafting operations, Delaney and co-workers found no differences in the incidences of ischemia (as measured by ECG changes) and few differences in other indices of myocardial oxygen demand.[17] As a result, these authors could not state, after carefully studying 16 patients, which agent resulted in more favorable myocardial oxygenation. They did hypothesize that in low concentrations, enflurane might be preferable to halothane in patients with severe ventricular dysfunction because of a greater decrease in systemic vascular resistance and thus afterload and a lesser increase in pulmonary capillary wedge pressure (increase in preload, which also increases myocardial oxygen demand). Unfortunately as of this date this hypothesis has not been adequately tested.

B. Induction of Anesthesia

Perhaps the single greatest advantage of the modern high dose opioid techniques now frequently employed for patients with CAD undergoing coronary artery bypass grafting (CABG) operations is the ability of these agents to rapidly induce profound analgesia and anesthesia without significantly affecting cardiovascular dynamics.[1-5] This is of particular importance during anesthetic induction. With large "anesthetic" doses of fentanyl,, significant hypotension and severe bradycardia are rare. Nonetheless, some clinicians have difficulties recognizing when patients are unconscious. Frequently, patients who appear to be unconscious have vigorous eyelid reflexes which are confusing to the anesthetist inexperienced with opioids. This is quite different from inhalation anesthetics, which clearly depress all reflexes and make the end point of anesthetic induction much easier to determine, even for the uninitiated and inexperienced anesthetist.

While speed of anesthetic induction is necessarily slower with inhalation anesthetics used without supplements, an appropriate ultra short acting intravenous induction agent employed shortly before or after allowing patients to breathe halothane, isoflurane or enflurane makes this type of induction as fast as any other. The real potential problem with induction of anesthesia with inhalation anesthetics is the lack of profound analgesia during endotracheal intubation and the resulting tachycardia and hypertension. This can be overcome by insuring that patients are well anesthetized (have sufficient concentrations of the inhalation agent on board to produce tracheal analgesia). However, adequate concentrations of inhalation anesthesia require time. But is an anesthetic induction which takes 5-10 minutes instead of 1-2 really that slow, especially if the result is greater hemodynamic stability?

Alternatively, induction of anesthesia with inhalation anesthetics can be very rapid with little risk of hemodynamic instability prior to and following endotracheal intubation, by employing 5-10 ug/kg of fentanyl followed by 1-1.5 mg/kg of sodium thiopental or etomidate (0.1-0.2 mg/kg) while the patient is breathing a tolerable concentration of halothane, enflurane or isoflurane. After paralysis with succinylcholine and endotracheal intubation, the inhalation anesthetic concentration is adjusted to maintain arterial blood pressures at desired levels. A slightly different technique which is especially useful in patients with CAD undergoing CABG operations is the use of high doses of fentanyl (25-40 ug/kg) plus oxygen for anesthetic induction and intubation followed by appropriate concentrations of the inhalation anesthetic. Advantages of this approach are a rapid, hemodynamicly event-free anesthetic induction, less possibility of cardiovascular depression (which will occasionally occur with thiopental or etomidate when they are given with or shortly after fentanyl) and less need for high concentrations of the potent inhalation agent during the maintenance phase of the anesthetic.

Induction with inhalation agents without supplements can be accomplished in patients with CAD undergoing CABG operations equally easily with isoflurane, enflurane or halothane. Recent studies suggest that if isoflurane is the agent of choice that induction is most rationally conducted by allowing patients to spontaneously ventilate for the first few moments, and then gradually taking over ventilation so that it becomes controlled shortly thereafter. The reason for this is that patients subjected to controlled ventilation are less likely to experience increases in arterial $PaCO_2$.[21] As a result cardiac output will remain unchanged, arterial blood pressure will decrease slightly (because of a decrease in peripheral resistance) and heart rate will only increase a small amount. When patients are allowed to breathe spontaneously and thus have elevated $PaCO_2$ (because of isoflurane induced respiratory depression), the cardiovascular respose to isoflurane is somewhat different. In these patients heart rate and cardiac output are frequently markedly increased.[21] These respiratory changes appear to be much more significant with isoflurane than halothane or enflurane.

Muscle Relaxants

Muscle relaxants are used for facilitating tracheal intubation, providing intercostal muscle paralysis so that sternal spread is less traumatic, preventing movements during light levels of anesthesia, eliminating diaphragmatic muscle movements and allowing controlled mechanical ventilation during CABG operations for patients with CAD. Although new short acting non-depolarizing muscle relaxants are about to be released and will undoubtedly change the practice of anesthesiologists, the most common muscle relaxants in use today are pancuronium, d-tubocurarine, dimethyltubocurarine, and succinylcholine. The most popular of these agents used for endotracheal intubation are succinylcholine and pancuronium while d-tubocurarine, dimethyltubocurarine and pancuronium are all frequently employed during maintenance of anesthesia.

The rational use of inhalation anesthetics for patients with coronary artery disease dictates that muscle relaxants also be employed with forethought and care. Since all of these agents can produce cardiovascular changes, their selection for use in specific patients should be dictated by that patient's previous medication history, specific premedication, and planned anesthetic drug sequence during both induction and maintenance. It makes little sense to employ agents or use techniques that multiply the chance for detrimental changes in hemodynamics. An example of this would be a patient having anesthesia induced with sodium thiopental, being paralyzed with a large dose of pancuronium for endotracheal intubation and having isoflurane as the maintenance anesthetic. Each of these agents is capable of increasing heart rate and pancuronium when administered as a large bolus may also increase arterial blood pressure,[22] particularly after a rapid sequence induction with sodium thiopental without use of an analgesic (Stanley TH, unpublished data).

In patients with CAD the use of a large dose of pancuronium for endotracheal intubation is rarely indicated because of the possibility of tachycardia and hypertension. A possible exception might be the patient receiving large doses of beta-blocking drugs preoperatively and subjected to a high dose narcotic induction sequence. The latter technique can result in significant bradycardia[23] and some clinicials reason that use of a large dose of pancuronium is effective in preventing this change.[24,25] Unfortunately, a large dose of pancuronium may overwhelm any narcotic induced bradycardia and result in tachycardia.[22,24] For this reason in employing narcotics for anesthetic induction, particularly before use of inhalaiton maintenance anesthesia, we use a belladonna premedication (to prevent bradycardia) and employ succinylcholine for endotracheal intubation.[23] Similarly the use of large doses of pancuronium following endotracheal intubation is also irrational, for similar reasons (potential of tachycardia and/or hypertension), and especially in patients having isoflurane anesthesia. Rather a more rational approach, at least from the cardiovascular point of view, would be to administer the drug in small (1-2 mg) increments until the desired level of muscle relaxation is achieved.

Following endotracheal intubation during maintenance inhalation anesthesia with halothane, enflurane or isoflurane, a large bolus of pancuronium may be quite desirable in patients who, for whatever reason, tend to have lower than desirable heart rates and arterial blood pressures and should be used in this situation. On the other hand, a much more rational approach in a patient with hypertension, tachycardia and an elevated cardiac output would be a large dose of d-tubocurarine (30 mg, perhaps given in divided doses) or dimethyltubocurarine. Even in patients with acceptable hemodynamics use of the curare like drugs may be more advantageous than a sympathomimetic like pancuronium if, for example, hemodynamics are on the high side of normal and a particularly stressful surgical stimulus is soon to occur.

Pancuronium and succinylcholine, as well as gallamine (a neuromuscular blocking agent not frequently used in CABG operations), result in more profound neuromuscular blockade in humans anesthetized with isoflurane than an equi-potent dose of halothane or nitrous oxide plus narcotic compounds.[26,27] For example, the median effective dose of pancuronium necessary to produce 50 percent depression of twitch height was 0.27 mg//m^2 during isoflurane anesthesia and 0.49 mg/m^2 during halothane anesthesia.[28] Similarly, curare is more potent in the presence presence of isoflurane than halothane.[29]

Maintenance of Anesthesia

It is clear that whether or not they are used during induction of anesthesia, inhalation anesthetics are frequently used in patients with CAD undergoing CABG operations during maintenance phases of the anesthetic technique.[1,17,22] Although it is impossible to exactly determine which of the inhalation agents available is most popular, it is clear that all are used and that while some clinicians use them without supplementation, most add narcotics to reduce inhalation requirements and a multiplicity of other agents to help optimize myocardial and peripheral vascular hemodynamics.[1,22] Some clinicians feel strongly that mixing opioids and other supplements with inhalation agents is the most rational approach to patients with CAD undergoing CABG operations. They cite that opioids and beta blockers can result in easier control of heart rate.[15,30] They add that selective use of nitrates, beta blockers, calcium blockers, nitroglycerin, alpha-adrenergic agonists and similar compounds are most effective in optimizing arterial blood pressure, myocardial contractility, left and right ventricular pre- and afterload, pulmonary and systemic vascular resistances and cardiac output and, therefore, are the best way of providing the ideal depth of anesthesia and protection to the heart.[15,30] Furthermore, they advocate that with one or more of the above that titration of the inhalation agent "to effect" is extremely easy and, therefore, that recovery can be rapid, if that is desirable (early extubation) or slower (more opioid --- later extubation). These are valid comments and taken in the broadest sense very desirable. However, one problem with this approach is that it leads to maximal polypharmacy and the potential for many drug interactions.

This author tends to be much more of a pharmacologic purist. Thus, when I mix opioids and inhalation agents, I try to avoid the use of other cardiovascularly acting drugs if at all possible. This can be done by increasing the dose of the opioid (usually fentanyl) and/or changing the concentration of the inahalation agent (usually isoflurane) to create the ideal pharmacological and physiological "atmosphere". Consequently, if systemic vascular resistance is a problem, blood pressure is adequate and the patient sufficiently anesthetized, the logical choice is a higher concentration of isoflurane which is an ideal "inhalation vasodilator" even in low concentrations and during cardiopulmonary bypass. Usually the result is that cardiac output (or flow) remains unchanged and resistance is rapidly decreased without the risk of "over shoot" so common with many of the intravenous vasodilators. While it is not always possible to simply use opioids and inhalation anesthetics, for example, with severe atrial tachycardias, it often is, and the result is an appropriate effect and an easier to understand pharmacologic picture. It is also important to emphasize that inhalation and intravenous anesthetics may produce serious cardiovascular, respiratory and other organ system problems when mixed with many of the popular supplements, i.e. significant and perhaps prolonged cardiovascular depression when mixed with the calcium channel blockers.[31] Therefore, in this author's opinion the simplest, most drug free technique that gets the job done is the best.

Conclusion

The skill of the anesthesiologist and his or her understanding of the pathology, the operation, and specific pharmacology and physiology are more important than the choice of any specific anesthetic agent or technique in patients with CAD undergoing CABG operations. Nonetheless, inhalation anesthetics do possess certain characteristics that make them highly desirable as anesthetics in these patients. Not the least of these qualities is ease of use and speed of onset. These two factors are probably the principal reason that intra-operative "awareness" is a much less frequent problem in patients being anesthetized with a potent inhalation anesthetic than when they are not.[32-34] Ease of producing myocardial depression (and reducing myocardial oxygen consumption) and decreasing central sympathetic output are always obvious advantages. Of course the fact that inhalation agents can be rapidly exhaled is another advantage in patients where a rapid recovery is desirable. It appears that for most clinicians these advantages when combined with those of intravenous agents, including those with and without anesthetic-analgesic actions, are important. Perhaps they are an important reason why coronary artery bypass operations are reasonably successful (low mortality and morbidity) and fairly simple anesthetic challenges for most active cardiac anesthesiologists. However, the one element of caution that must be appreciated when this approach is employed is the possibility of dangerous drug interaction. Unfortunately, drug interaction is often difficult to appreciate and terminate when large numbers of drugs are employed.

REFERENCES

1. Wynands JE, Townsend GE, Ping Wong BS, et al: Blood pressure response and plasma fentanyl concentrations during high and very high dose fentanyl anesthesia for coronary artery surgery. Anesth Analg 62:661-665, 1983
2. Kono K, Philbin DM, Coggins CH, et al: Renal function and stress response during halothane or fentanyl anesthesia. Anesth Analg 60:552-556, 1981
3. Lunn JK, Stanley TH, Eisele J, et al: High dose fentanyl anesthesia for coronary artery surgery: Plasma fentanyl concentrations and influence of nitrous oxide on cardiovascular responses. Anesth Analg 58:390-395, 1979
4. Preston TA: Coronary artery surgery: A critical review. Raven Press, New York, 1977
5. Watanabe E, Covell JW, Marko PR, et al: The effects of increased arterial pressures and positive inotropic agents on the severity of myocardial ischemia in the acutely depressed heart. Am J Cardiolog 30:371-377, 1972
6. Braunwald E: The determinants of myocardial oxygen consumption. Physiologist 12:65-93, 1969
7. Waller JL: Anesthesia for coronary revascularization. In Kaplan JA: Cardiac Anesthesia, Clinical Cardiology Monographs, Grune and Stratton, New York, 1979, p 241
8. Bland JHL, Lowenstein E: Halothane-induced decrease in experimental myocardial ischemia in the non-failing canine heart. Anesthesiology 45:387-293, 1976
9. Merin RG: Effect of anesthetics on the heart. Surg Clin North Am 55:759-774, 1975

10. Shimosato S, Etsten BE: Effects of anesthetic drugs on the heart: A critical review of myocardial contractility and its relation to hemodynamics. Clin Anesth 3:17-72, 1969

11. Eger EI, Smith NT, Stoelting RK, et al: Cardiovascular effects of halothane in man. Anesthesiology 32:396-409, 1970

12. Levesque PR, Nanagas V, Shanks C, et al: Circulatory effects of enflurane in normocarbic human volunteers. Can Anaesth Soc J 21: 580-585, 1974

13. Stevens WC, Cromwell TH, Halsey MH, et al: Cardiovascular effects of a new inhalation anesthetic, Forane, in human volunteers at constant arterial carbon dioxide tension. Anesthesiology 35:8-16, 1971

14. Merin RG, Kumazawa T, Luka NL: Enflurane depresses myocardial function, perfusion, and metabolism in the dog. Anesthesiology 45:501-507, 1976

15. Waller JL, Kaplan JA, Jones EL: Anesthesia for coronary revascularization, in Kaplan JA: Cardiac Anesthesia, Clinical Cardiology Monographs, Grune and Stratton, New York, 1979, pp 241-280

16. Hamilton WK: Do let the blood pressure drop and do use myocardial depressants! Anesthesiology 45:273-274, 1976

17. Delaney TJ, Kistner JR, Lake CL, et al: Myocardial function during halothane and enflurane anesthesia in patients with coronary artery disease. Anesth Analg 59:240-244, 1980

18. Eger EI II: Isoflurane: A review. Anesthesiology 55:559-576, 1981

19. Johnston RR, Eger EI II, Wilson CL: A comparative interaction of epinephrine with enflurane, isoflurane and halothane in man. Anesth Analg (Cleve) 55:709-712, 1976

20. Tarnow J, Eberlein HJ, Oser G, et al: Influence of modern inhalation anesthetics on haemodynamics, myocardial contractility, left ventricular volumes and myocardial oxygen supply. Anaesthetist 26:220-230, 1977

21. Cromwell TH, Stevens WC, Eger EI II, et al: The cardiovascular effects of compound 469 (Forane) during spontaneous ventilation and CO_2 challenge in man. Anesthesiology 35:17-25, 1971

22. Waller JL, Hug CC Jr, Nagle DM, et al: Hemodynamic changes during fentanyl-oxygen anesthesia for aorto-coronary bypass operation. Anesthesiology 55:212-217, 1981

23. Stanley TH, Philbin DM, Coggins CH: Fentanyl-oxygen anesthesia for coronary artery surgery: Cardiovascular and anti-diuretic hormone responses. Can Anaesth Soc J 26:168-172, 1979

24. Sebel PS, Bovill GJ, Boekhorst RAA, et al: Cardiovascular effects of high dose fentanyl anesthesia. Acta Anesthesiol Scand 26:308-315, 1982

25. Wynands JE, Wong P, Whalley DG, et al: Wxygen fentanyl anesthesia and plasma fentanyl concentrations in patients with poor left ventricular function. Anesth Analg 62:476-482, 1983

26. Ali HH, Savarese JJ: Monitoring of neuromuscular function. Anesthesiology 45:216-249, 1976

27. Stevens WC, Cromwell TH, Halsey MJ, et al: The cardiovascular effects of a new inhalation anesthetic, Forane, in human volunteers at constant arterial carbon dioxide tension. Anesthesiology 35:8-16, 1971

28. Miller RD, Way WL, Dolan WM, et al: Comparative neuromuscular effects of pancuronium, gallamine and succinylcholine during Forane and halothane anesthesia in man. Anesthesiology 35:509-514, 1971
29. Miller RD, Eger EI II, Way WL, et al: Comparative neuromuscular effects of Forane and halothane alone and in combination with d-tubocurarine in man. Anesthesiology 35:38-42, 1971
30. Thomas SJ: Anesthesia considerations for coronary revascularization. In ASA Refresher Course Lectures, Oct. 1982, p 201
31. Reves JG: Calcium channel blockers and anesthesia. In New Anesthetic Agents, Devices and Monitoring Techniques, edited by Stanley TH and Petty WC, Martin Nijhoff, The Hague, 1983, pp 67-76
32. Brice DD, Hetherington RR, Utting JE: A simple study of awareness and dreaming during anaesthesia. Br J Anaesth 42:535-542, 1970
33. Wong KC, Martin WE, Hornbein TF, et al: The cardiovascular effects of morphine sulfate with oxygen and with nitrous oxide in man. Anesthesiology 38:542-549, 1973
34. Knight PR, Pandit SK, Bolles R, et al: Amnesia to visual stimulation after large doses of fentanyl. Anesthesiology 53:S2, 1980

PREVENTION, RECOGNITION AND MANAGEMENT OF INTRAOPERATIVE
MYOCARDIAL ISCHEMIA

JOHN H. TINKER, M.D.

THE "EPIDEMIOLOGY"

Approximately 600,000 American will die this year of coronary
artery disease (CAD) and its related complications. About 1.3 million
people in the United States suffer a new myocardial infarction (MI)
each year. Over 4 million people in this country are alive who have
experienced at least one prior MI. One estimate has it that ± 40
million Americans have some degree of coronary artery disease.[1] Therefore, having to anesthetize someone with one or other form of this
epidemic disease is a near-daily occurrence in most anesthesia practices. Assessment of the risk involved allows more informed decision
making relative to whether or not to proceed with surgery in the first
place, and it allows decisions as to invasive monitoring, choice of
anesthetic technique, postoperative management, to be at least somewhat
more informed.

THE RISK

Topkins and Artusio reported in 1964 that the risk of anesthesia
and surgery was many fold increased if the patient had suffered a prior
MI.[2] Tarhan et al,[3] in 1972, in a study of approximately 35,000 patients,
reported that risk of perioperative* MI was about 6% if the patient had
had a prior MI vs 0.13% if the patient had not. Further, they reported
that if the prior MI had occurred within three months, the risk was 37%;
between three to six months, 16%. In addition, the mortality of such a
perioperative reinfarction was 50%. In 1978 Steen et al[4] reported on a
series of 73,000 patients of who 587 had suffered a documented prior MI.
Again, the overall risk of 6% was evident, also with similar high risk
for patients with 3 months (27%) and within 3-6 months (11%) of an
* Usually defined as an MI occurring within seven days of anesthesia
and surgery.

infarct. In this report, death occurred 69% of the time. The contention by Steen et al[4] that little if any imporvement in this problem had occurred between 1968 and 1975 (in the same institution) was met with two basic kinds of criticisms. First, critics said, "We know we're doing better than that in our institution." In fact, since those reports, with the prospective exception to be mentioned below, no reports of improved results have been published. Secondly, critics said, "Your problem lies postoperatively, not intraoperatively--it is the surgeons who are not taking adequate postoperative care of these patients." Actually, 9 of 36 perioperative infarctions in the report by Steen et al[4] occurred during anesthesia and surgery. Besides, why should any expertise possessed by anesthesiologists not be applied postoperatively as well? In other words, if postoperative management is at fault then we in anesthesia must shoulder some of the blame. In late 1980, Eerola et al[5] performed the same type of study, again retrospectively, and reported essentially the same overall 6% risk figure, and similar high risk for anesthesia and surgery in patients with a recent MI.

These are retrospective studies, and as such have both benefits and drawbacks. They do "tell it like it is", in the sense that actual performance can be examined without the people involved "tightening up their practices". Their obvious drawback is not so much in their lack of controls as it is in their lack of detailed consistent documentation. The lack of proper control groups is obvious, and it prevents anything more than speculation as to causes of the observed phenomena. Still, as long as retrospective studies are only used to record incidences they can be very useful. For example, the above studies convinced most physicians to postpone truly elective surgery six months after an MI. Few would argue with this today. There is danger in the uncritical acceptance of a study which claims to be "prospective". First, if the individuals whose practice is being monitored know that that is the case, they may, consciously or not, modify that practice in ways which could easily influence the outcome. The interested reader is referred to a paper by Radford et al,[6] which documents this phenomenon very well.

The other problem with some "prospective" studies is that, in fact, they are not really prospective. The paper by Goldman et al[7] is a case in point. The authors performed histories and physicals preoperatively, and then very carefully followed the patients' post-operative course, looking for cardiac morbidity and correlating it with preoperative history, physical, and lab findings. The study is extremely useful and important, but despite the word in its title, it is not prospective. No attempt was made to influence either choice of timing or anesthesia and surgery. The study is merely "immediate retrospective" with the better documentation that implies, as opposed to "remote retrospective" e.g. the study by Steen et al.[4] Goldman et al[7] established an elaborate point scoring system which correlated with their retrospectivly determined cardiac risk. They added S-3 gallop, neck vein distention, and many other evidences of decreased contrac-tility to prior MI as risk factors. The point scale they constructed has proved unwieldy and is not widely used today. Further, no truly prospective studies of the risk using their point scale have validated it. Still, studies such as Goldman et al[7] do represent important attempts to document and quantify risk in the commonly-seen patients.

What about the patient with hypertension? Steen et al[4] reported that hypertension in patients with a prior MI, defined only as that diagnosis having been entered somewhere in the record, resulted in a doubling of the perioperative infarction rate. Goldman et al,[8] in a distinct communication from the above, but using the same data base, could not find evidence that preoperative hypertension added to peri-operative risk. Prys-Roberts,[9] in an accompanying editorial, pointed out that the patients of Goldman et al[8] were, for the most part, adequately treated, and that the report should not be construed as permission to proceed with anesthesia in a patient with relatively unchecked hypertension if the surgery is at all elective.

Patients who have survived prior coronary artery bypass grafting (CABG) are frequently encountered, scheduled for subsequent surgery of all types. Mahar et al[10] reported on 99 of these patients who underwent a total of 168 subsequent non-cardiac operations. Not a single perioperative MI occurred. This either means that CABG was efficacious in preventing subsequent MI, or the CABG constituted a "survival test", i.e. that the perioperative MI that was "waiting to happen" happened during or after The CABG, and was not "available" to happen after the next operation! Whatever the explanation, the clinically relevant point is that patients scheduled for surgery after CABG seem not to be nearly as great a risk as those who have suffered prior MI.

Backer et al[11] studied over 10,000 patients who underwent ophthalmic operations using local and/or retrobulbar block anesthesia, with anesthesia personnel in attendance and recording blood pressures, etc. Well documented MI's had occurred prior to 288 of these operations (in 195 patients). Again, not a single perioperative reinfarction occurred. This does not indicate local to be safer than general anesthesia, but again the clinically relevant point is that patients with prior MI presenting for opthalmic operations under local anesthesia seem to constitute a trivial risk.

Other aspects of the risk problem include length of surgery, patient age and sex, site and type of operation, presence of diabetes and thyroid disease. Steen et al[4] reported a striking correlation between length of surgery and perioperative infarction incidence. More detailed multifactorial analysis indicates that length of surgery influences perioperative MI risk only for operations on thorax, great vessels, or upper abdomen lasting longer than three hours. Site of surgery was also important. The three above mentioned locations were the only ones associated with significantly greater incidences of perioperative infarction than the overall group. There were no detectable sex differences, nor could diabetes be singled out retrospectively. Incidence of perioperative infarction increased numerically but not statistically with advancing age. General was neither safer nor less safe than major regional anesthesia.[4]

To briefly summarize, much is known about perioperative risk in patients with CAD. If they are going to succumb shortly after surgery, it is overwhelmingly likely to be due to an MI or some cardiac complication, rather than some complicaton of the operation itself. It seems very likely that nearly 6 percent of patients with prior MI still have another MI during or just following anesthesia and surgery, and half of these will die. It is still true that elective surgery should be postponed after MI for six months unless that surgery is a coronary artery bypass. It is also true that anesthesiologists ought to participate actively in these decisions.

THE PROPRANOLOL BUSINESS

Many CAD patients take propranolol or other beta blocker. Viljoen et al,[12] in 1972 concluded that propranolol should be discontinued well prior to anesthesia and surgery. A massive literature refutes that today, and few anesthesiologist would either taper or discontinue the drug prior to _any_ surgery now. Still, we do often stop propranolol _during_ and _after_ the surgery. We very carefully titrate our diabetic patients with respect to their insulin dosage re: urine and/or blood sugars perioperatively, but we allow our propranololized patients who are NPO to remain off the drug postoperatively, sometimes for many days. Perhaps this is a contributing cause to the continued high incidence of perioperative MI.

HYPOTHERMIA[13]

How many times have you entered an OR and found the anesthesia personnel wrapped in a blanket? Hypothermia patients with CAD (known or unsuspected) who awaken after anesthesia with shivering may experience a 200-500 percent increase in whole body oxygen demand, just the sort of thing that might set up the condition for a perioperative MI, and just the sort of clinical care item we can relatively easily improve.

PAIN

Postoperative patients are often forced to suffer greater pain than really necessary. Physicians' narcotic orders often border on the homeopathic. Nurses are well aware of the dangers of unattended narcotized older patients and so often give less than the maximal PRN ordered dose and at longer intervals. Severe pain and anxiety, with attendant tachycardia and increased arterial pressure may again be contributory to conditons just right for perioperative MI. In the average busy practice, postoperative analgesia is seldom, if ever, the province of anyone remotely expert in pain management. Certainly our care can be improved in this area. Perhaps an added benefit would be fewer MI's. On the other hand, a relatively hypovolemic patient, given narcotics, who develops hypotension, who already has CAD-related pressure dependent coronary blood flow, may be set up for this MI if hypotension is allowed to persist.

PREOPERATIVE CARDIAC ASSESSMENT

Besides the history (prior MI, angina), what predictors of outcome can we find that are clinically obtainable and relevant? Many of these patients (with documented CAD) have undergone catheterization and coronary angiography. If not, and you have any reason to suspect serious CAD, you should consider the fact that in competent laboratories the risk of coronary angiography is less than 0.1 percent, and perhaps postpone elective surgery accordingly. Certainly someone who is having "angina" out in the hall awaiting a total hip reeplacement should not be anesthetized until a full ECG has been read by a qualified MD and incipient MI has been ruled out.

Cath reports will have several numbers of use to anesthesiologist. Left ventricular end-diastolic pressure, if greater than 15 mm HG, indicates a ventricle with little reserve and poor contractility, as does an ejection fraction less than 50 percent. Left main coronary stenosis of >50% means a potential anesthetic disaster and should raise all sorts of red flags. "Right coronary dominance" means only that the coronary supplies and AV node and should not distract you from the conditon of the left main coronary. Patients with mitral insufficiency (two "outlets" from the left ventricle) may have misleadingly high ejection fractions, i.e. their contractility may in fact not be that good. Similarly, patients with aortic stenosis or LV aneurysm may have lower ejection fractions than would be the case withou the obstruction to outflow in the aortic stenosis of the aneurysmal sac in the latter case. Ejection fraction, very useful in estimateing cardiac difficulties durng anesthesia, must be interpreted intelligently. Ejection fraction is correlated with survival, both in medical and CABG treated groups of patients with CAD. Newer echocardiographic and angiographic assessment of regional ventricular wall motion may allow us to be much more accurate in pinpointing individual preoperative high risk patients.

CAN WE DO BETTER?

Rao and El etr,[14] in 1981, reported on 97 patients who had documented MI within the previous six months who underwent anesthesia and surgery. REinfarction rate for patients with MI less than three months old was 7.8%, with postoperative mortality 5.3%. A 3.4% infarction rate was reported inpatients with prior MI's three to six months old.

They attributed their reduction of the prior risk results to intensive intra- and postoperative invasive hemodynamic monitoring, with aggressive treatments of aberrations continuing postoperatively. This report, if it can be confirmed, is very encouraging, for it provides justification for such increasingly popular practices, but more importantly, may represent a real advance in the care of these patients.

REFERENCES

1. Preston TA. Coronary artery surgery: a critical review. New York, Raven Press 1977.
2. Topkins MJ, Artusio JF. Myocardial infarction and surgery, a five year study. Anesth Analg 1964;23:716.
3. Tarhan S, Moffitt EA, Taylor WF, et al. Myocardial infarction after general anesthesia. JAMA 1972;220:1451.
4. Steen PA, Tinker JH, TArhan S. Myocardial reinfarction after anesthesia and surgery. JAMA 1978;239:2566.
5. Eerola M, Eerola R, Kaukinen S, Kaukinen L. Risk factors in surgical patients with varied preoperative myocardial infarction. ACTA Anaesth Scand 1980;24:219-223.
6. Little JB, Radford EP. Effects of ionizing radiation and their importance in anesthesiology. Anesthesiology 1964;25:479-489.
7. Goldman L, Caldera DL, Nussbaum SB, et al. Multifactorial index of cardiac risk in noncardiac surgical procedures. N Engl J Med 1977;197:845.
8. Goldman L, Caldera DL. Risks of general anesthesia and elective operation in the hypertensive patient. Anesthesiology 1979;50:285-292.
9. Prys-Roberts C. Hypertension and anesthesia--fifty years on. Editorial. Anesthesiology 1979;50:281-284.
10. Mahar LJ, Steen PA, Tinker JH, et al. Perioperative myocardial infarction in patients with coronary artery disease with and without aorta-coronary artery bypass grafts. J Thor Cardiovasc Surg 1978; 26:533.
11. Backer CL, Tinker JH, Robertson DM, Vlietstra RE. Myocardial reinfarction following local anesthesia and ophthalmic surgery. Anesth Analg 1980;59:257-262.
12. Viljoen JF, Estafanous FG, Kellner GA. Propranolol and cardiac surgery. J Thor Cardiovasc Surg 1972;64:826.
13. Noback CR, Tinker JH. Hypothermia after cardiopulmonary bypass in man: amelioration by nitroprusside-induced vasodilation during rewarming. Anesthesiology 1980;53:277-280.
14. Rao TLK, El Etr AA. Myocardial reinfarction following anesthesia in patients with recent infarctions. Proceedings, 55th Congress Int Anes REs Soc, Atlanta. March 1981, pp 131-132

OTHER SUGGESTED READINGS

1. Braunwald E, Ross J Jr, Sonnenblick EH. Mechanisms of contraction in the normal and failing heart. Boston, Little, Brown Co., 1976.
2. Brown BR. Anesthesia dn the patient with heart disease. Philadelphia, F.A. Davis Co., 1980.
3. Kaplan JA: Cardiac anesthesia. New York, Grune and Stratton, 1979.
4. Shepherd JT, Vanhoutte PM. The human cardiovascular system, facts and concepts. New York, Raven Press, 1979.
5. Branthwaite MA. Anaesthesia for cardiac surgery and allied procedure. London, Blackwell Scientific Publications, 1980.

ANESTHETIC MANAGEMENT OF CHILDREN WITH CONGENITAL HEART DISEASE

ALVIN HACKEL,M.D.

Preparations for the intraoperative care of a child about to undergo cardiac surgery begin with the preoperative visit of the anesthesiologist. In addition to the material discussed in the previous lecture on this subject, the appropriate preoperative medication must be considered. As previously noted, the chronic anxiety of the patient can only be partially alleviated by a carefully conducted preoperative visit. Nevertheless, preoperative medication is essential in this group of patients.

Preoperative medication is recommended in all but the most unusual circumstances for pediatric cardiac patients weighing more than 10 kg or who are more than one year of age. We recommend the use of a moderately heavy premedication, usually a narcotic administered intramuscularly. Because of concern about hypoventilation secondary to the use of these drugs, their administration should be planned so the child is in the operating room suite, and under the surveillance of the anesthesia team, before the time of maximum drug effect.

Maintenance of the physiologic status quo and/or an increase in systemic oxygenation are the anesthesiologist's goals for the anesthesia induction phase. Children with borderline oxygenation and perfusion will have a chronic metabolic acidosis, an increased systemic vascular resistance, and a minimal cardiac reserve. The choice of anesthetic(s) to be used for induction is determined by correlating the pathophysiology of the cardiac abnormalities present and the advantages and disadavantages of the agents under consideration. The choice is between ketamine, narcotics, and inhalation agents. Each one can be used safely. There is a difference, however, in the margin of safety offered between the various anesthetics. Ketamine is, for the majority of pediatric cardiac cases, the current drug of choice for induction. The summation of its effects on the cardiovascular system is a protection of the left-to-right shunting which occurs so frequently in this group of patients. It prevents the reversal of these shunts which occur with a decrease in systemic vascular resistance and/or a decrease in myocardial contractility. The newer narcotics in the fentanyl family are popular because of their benign effects on the cardiovascular system.

The intent of pediatric cardiovascular monitoring is to ensure optimal tissue perfusion through careful observation of the systems involved. The simplest techniques are the precordial stethescope, digital palpation of the peripheral pulse, visual evaluation of the skin color and tissue perfusion, and visual evaluation of cardiac function when the thoracic cavity is open. More complex techniques include the cuff and Doppler blood pressure measurements, the ECG, and finger pulse plethysmography. The most complex techniques are on-line monitoring of arterial and central venous pressure. The intent is to utilize the best tools available to acquire the information needed for patient management.

Placing indwelling arterial and central venous catheters in pediatric patients is often viewed with trepidation by anesthesiologists who do not care for infants and children on a regular basis. With proper technique, the insertion of an arterial catheter in a pediatric patient is associated with a high success rate. The chosen extremity is immobilized. The artery is then palpated with one hand and the catheter inserted with the other at a 45 degree angle into and through the artery (Fig. 1). With the stylus of the catheter at least partially removed, the catheter is withdrawn slowly and then when there is a pulsating flow of blood from the catheter, it is pushed forward in the artery. The tubing is then attached to the catheter and the catheter is secured in place. Multiple attempts may be necessary to accomplish the catheterization. More than one site may have to be tried. The most frequent arteries used are the radial arteries. If cannulation of a more peripheral artery cannot be accomplished, a femoral artery can be cannulated with the same type of needle/catheter/wire system used for central venous cannulation.

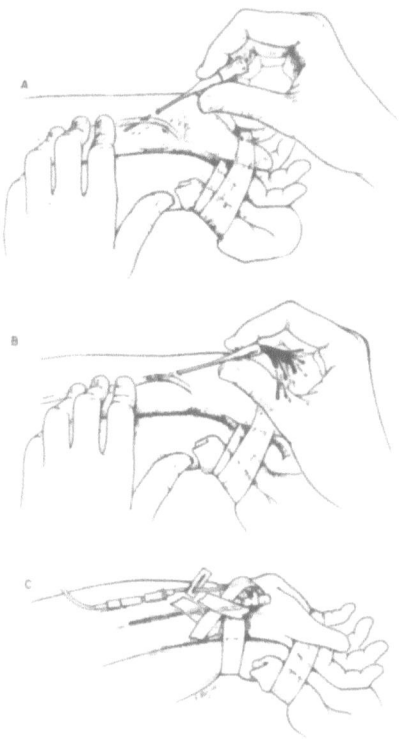

Figure 1. Radial artery cannulation. (Ream AK, Fogdall,
RP, eds. Anesthetic Management of the Pediatric
Patient. In Acute Cardiovascular Management.
Philadelphia, JB Lippincott)

The insertion of a central venous catheter is usually
achieved by cannulation of an external or internal jugular
vein. The cannulation technique for pediatric patients is
no different than that of adults. The landmarks are usually
easier to palpate, although they are closer together.

Temperature monitoring is important in all pediatric
patients and particularly so in cardiac patients because of
the inclusion of hypothermia as part of the surgical

management in this group of patients. Both the rectal and
esophageal temperatures should be measured continuously.
The airway temperature should also be monitored when a
heated humidified anesthesia circuit is used.

The management of intraoperative fluid therapy in the
pediatric cardiac patient can be difficult. The maintenance
fluid volume required is a small quantity; drugs must be
given and flushed through intravenous lines, and the
patency of the intra-arterial catheter must be maintained.
The composition of the intravenous fluid is not of great
importance for the older pediatric patient. Five percent
dextrose/0.225 percent normal saline is recommended as a
maintenance solution. A ten percent dextrose parenteral
solution is recommended for infants. The infusion rate
depends on the volume state of the patient.

Management of cardiopulmonary bypass does not differ
significantly between pediatric and adult patients, except
perhaps for the greater application of the "primacy of flow
principle" as contrasted to the concept of maintaining the
mean arterial pressure at a level of at least 75 mm Hg.

In the immediate post-bypass period, special attention
should be paid to the volume status of the patient. Whole
blood can be administered more rapidly than packed red
blood cells through pediatric-sized intravenous catheters
and should be used for blood volume replacement.

There are many different "recipes" for inotropic drug
administration in the post-bypass period. Dopamine appears
to be the most frequently used agent to enhance myocardial

contractility, either temporarily because of coronary air, or in a more prolonged manner because of persistent anatomical or surgically acquired problems. The placement of pacemaker wires is essential after any complicated pediatric surgical repair. Chronotropic agents are difficult to titrate to effective levels.

The transition between the intra-operative and post-operative periods should be as smooth as possible. Preferably the anesthesiologist team will participate in the post-operative management of the patient. The individual patient management experience acquired in the operating room should be transmitted to the post-operative care team.

There should be no rush to move the pediatric patient through the post-operative management period. The principles are the same as those for adult post-operative care. Pediatric patients should remain intubated and receiving assisted ventilation until there is incontrovertible evidence that he or she can breathe spontaneously in a manner allowing for adequate ventilation and oxygenation without an inordinate percentage of their cardiac output being used for respiration.

As stated in the previous presentation on congenital heart disease, the strides made in the surgical and anesthetic management of congenital heart disease are one of the recent triumphs of modern medicine. With careful and appropriate management of these patients, a high percentage will leave the hospital and go on to lead lives compatible

98

with a relatively normal physiologic state. For the remainder who do not, the pursuit of further advances in this field continues.

1. Hackel A. Anesthetic Management of the Pediatric Patient, in Acute Cardiovascular Management, Ream AK, Fogdall RP(eds). Philadelphia, JB Lippincott, 1982.

2. Bland JW, Williams WH. Anesthesia for Treatment of Congenital Heart Defects, in Cardiac Anesthesia, Kaplan JA (ed). New York, Grune & Stratton, 1979.

3. Rogers MC, Smith RM. Anesthesia for intrathoracic and cardiac surgery, in Anesthesia for Infants and Children, Smith RM(ed). St. Louis, CV Mosby, 1980.

4. Loomis JC. Care of the Pediatric Patient following Cardiovascular Surgery, in Acute Cardiovascular Management, Ream AK, Fogdall RP(eds). Philadelphia, JB Lippincott, 1982.

TECHNICAL ASPECTS OF PERFORMANCE OF CARDIOPULMONARY BYPASS: THE PUMP
THE OXYGENATOR, PITFALLS, DISASTERS AND NUANCES

JOHN H. TINKER, M.D.

INTRODUCTION

I have been in an operating room wherein the perfusionist and the
anesthesiologist had little communication. The perfusionist had decided
that the arterial pressure should be 60 mm Hg, but the anesthesiologist
had decided it should be 70. The anesthesiologist would turn up his
phenylephrine drip and, shortly therafter, sure enough, the perfusionist
would turn down the pump flow! I believe that anesthesiologists should
understand cardiopulmonary bypass, from the standpoints of its routine
application and its use as a therapeutic tool during dire emergencies.
In this lecture, we will be discussing non pulsatile bypass almost
exclusively because that is the type in widespread use.

AVAILABLE CIRCUITS

First, it is necessary that anesthetist understand the kinds of
circuits that are available. Most commonly, flow s diverted from either
the venae cavae or the right atrium itself to the pump oxygenator and
thence back to the aorta. It is also possible to divert flow from the
femoral vein cannulation site (the cannula tip should be in the inferior
vena cava) back to the aorta. It is also possible to divert flow from
any of the above venous drainage sites and replace it at the femoral
artery. It is even possible to use the bracheal artery as an arterial
inflow site, but this is seldom done due to size limitations.

The usual circuit in use today is depicted in figure 1.

FIGURE 1

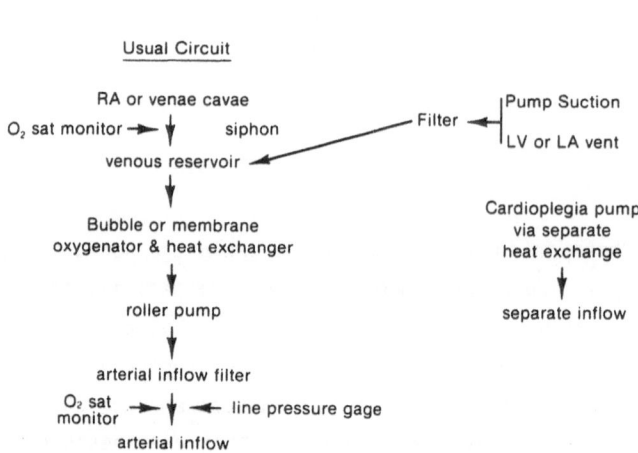

There are several things of special interest aobut this circuit. First, note that an <u>oxygen saturation monitor</u> can be placed on the venous outflow to the venous reservoir and also on the arterial inflow line. It is likely that in the near future an infrared device will be available which will allow the perfusionist to read PaO_2, $PaCO_2$, pHa, and inflowing perfusate temperature, all from the arterial inflow line itself. The device will use infrared fluorescence refractometry, and will not actually contact blood. Next, again referring to figure 1, note that the blood flowing via the venous drainage is in fact a siphon. No pumps are involved in this side of the circuit. It is very possible to have an "air lock" i.e., a disruption of the siphon by a large air bubble. This is especially likely during valvular complex congenital surgery wherein the right side of the heart is being operated upon. Surgical manuevering may disrupt the seal around the right atrial cannula, allowing air to enter the siphon. The anesthestist can provide early warning of this if it is recurring.

The roller pumps in use today are almost, but not quite, occlusive. The adjustment of tension on these pumps is a critical factor; the manufacturers recommendations must be followed closely. Note also that the roller pump in use today is powered by a "<u>constant speed</u>" electric motor. Most electric motors are inherently variable speed devices;

when changes in load are placed upon them, speed (therefore output) varies greatly. This is obviously an undesirable feature for a bypass pump. The pumps in use today are sophisticated <u>constant speed pumps</u> wherein the speed, once set, remains constant even if the pressure load changes over a fairly wide range. This is one factor in the high cost of these pumps.

Another factor regarding the quality of these pumps is the fact that they come equipped with line voltage variation protection circuits. If line voltage varies (over a reasonable range), i.e., a "brownout", pump speed and force will remain constant or nearly so. The pump can be cranked by hand incase of failure.

Again referring to figure 1, note that there is an <u>arterial inflow filter</u> in most circuits today. Microemboli, particulate matter from the cardiotomy suction, are removed by filtration--usually at 40u. There must be a bypass around this filter in case it becomes clogged to an important degree. The perfusionist must be able to instantly bypass this filter, should it become an obstacle.

The other roller pumps on the pump oxygenator are used for the following purposes: 1) cardioplegia infusion is usually done today by the perfusionist because large volumes of very cold solution need to be pumped as rapidly as possible. 2) There is almost uniform use today, if surgically possible, of a left ventricular venting device so as to never permit excessive distending pressure to be placed on the left ventricle. Today, this is usually placed via purse string suture through the right superior pulmonary vein, into the left atrium, through the mitral valve into the left ventricle. Some surgeons still perfer to place this vent throught he apex of the left ventricle (thus creating a small infarct). 3) The cardiotomy suction. With respect to use of the latter device, the perfusionist must not permit this suction to excessively traumatize blood by use of excessive speeds on the pump heads. A common phrase used in the past was that the perfusionnist would run the cardiotomy suction "by ear", the idea being that loud slurping noises were indicative of increased degrees of blood trauma. This seems good practice. Another important point about the cardiotomy suction; inexperienced surgical assistants, in their zeal to obtain as dry a field for the surgeon as possible, often use the "high power" or wall suction. Blood suction into this device is lost permanently unless a centrifugation-type blood washer is in use. The experienced anesthetist will caution the surgical assistants against excessive use of the "wall suction", making light of it sometimes if necessary but with a clear purpose in mind of saving the patient exogenous transfusion.

Again referring to figure 1, note the location of the "line pressure gauge". This is an important component of a safe cardiopulmonary bypass circuit and, unfortunately, is not in universal use throughout the United States. During bypass, this gauge usually reads 200 to 300 mm Hg, and represents the presure in the arterial inflow line, note the pressure in the arterial system of the patient. The arterial inflow line is quite small relative to the size of the aorta. Thus a large pressure differential across it is expected. It is entirely possible to have arterial inflow line pressures of 300 mm Hg while at the same time having a radial arterial pressure of less than 50 mm Hg. This line pressure is important for two reasons; 1) at pressures exceeding 300 to 350 mm Hg, there is reasonable danger that one or more of the high pressure fittings will explode, resulting in disaster; 2) after the aortic inflow line is placed in the aorta and the pump is attached to it, it is very important that the arterial line be opened and the perfusionist state clearly that he sees pulsations on the arterial inflow line pressure gauge. Absence of pulsations at this stage may indicate that the patient has been attached to the cardiopulmonary bypass circuit backwards! It is not impossible to attache the venous drainage line to the arterial inflow side and not know it because of a clamp that is always placed on the venous line. Careful attention to the presence of these pulsations will prevent this disaster. There is controversy amoung perfusionists about the necessity of having an arterial inflow line pressure gauge. I believe strongly in it, and have seen patients saved from disasters by it. Finally, when everything is thought to be ready to go on bypass and the surgeon says "on bypass" and the perfusionist starts the pumphead turning, the presence of arterial inflow line pressure gauge will tell him rapidly whether or not a clamp has been inadvertantly left on the arterial line in the surgical field. If this is the case, the arterial line inflow pressure will rise to dangerous levels and the pump technician will know to turn off the pump head and request said clamp to be removed. In the absence of such a pressure gauge, a rather spectacular explosion is likely next! In additon, presence of pulsations, during the period just before going on bypass, detected by the perfusionist on the arterial inflow line pressure gauge is a reasonable indication that the arterial inflow line has in fact been placed in the true lumen of the aorta. This can help prevent aortic dissection (see below).

BLOOD GAS MEASUREMENT ON BYPASS

Oxygen saturation devices, employing infrared, are on the market today and enable continuous measurement of oxygen saturation in both the arterial inflow and venous outflow sides of the circuit. As anesthesiologists, some of us can remember the days wherein oxygen saturation was all that we had available as well. When partial pressures of dissolved blood gases became available, we found them much more useful for our monitoring of these patients. I believe that the new devices, soon to be marketed, which will permit continuous online arterial and venous blood gases, at the actual temperature of the perfusate, will represent real advances. Currently, many centers still rely on intermittent blood gas sampling. This is potentially hazardous because oxygen requirements can change rapidly, especially during the rewarming period. Estimations of oxygen delivery requirements (pump flow) based on body size and temperature are notoriously inaccurate.

ANTICOAGULATION FOR BYPASS

First and foremost, please never administer heparin for anticoagulation for bypass except in a central line which has a freely flowing venous return. There is little if any excuse for ever administering heparin for anticoagulation for bypass into a peripheral i.v. This author knows of at least one case wherein the heparin was administered into a peripheral vein, but a blood pressure cuff proximally prevented very much if any of the heparin from entering the systemic circulation. The result was a clotted pump and death. If the intravenous line in which you are considering adminstering heparin is not funcitoning to your complete satisfaction, please ask the surgeon to administer heparin directly into the right atrium. many surgeons prefer to do this anyway and, given various mistakes of the past, one finds it hard to argue with them.

There is controversy regarding fixed dosage heparin i.e., 3 mg per kilo or 90 mg/m^2 versus the so called "dose response" method of administering heparin which involves the use of the activated coagulation time (ACT) and drawing a dose response curve. The theory behind the administration of any drug via a dose response method is sound if the response is consistent. The problem with the usually measured ACT's is that there is enough inconsistency for concern. The theory that administration of heparin by one of the fixed dosage schedules mentioned above might cause a small number of patients who have antithrombin-III deficiency to fail tobe completely anticoagulated, is not borne out be large centers with experience with many thousands of cases. Another often stated theory regarding this is that even if gross coagulation does not occur, these supposedly under-anticoagulated patients (with antithromin-III deficiency) will have microscopic clotting which will be deposited here and there. I also do not subscribe to this theory. I believe that fixed dose anticoagulation with heparin 90 mg/m^2 is a proven safe and effective method of anticoagulation for cardiopulmonary bypass. It is also extremely simple compared to the dose response methodology.

Once on bypass, do you administer more heparin? The activated coagulation time (ACT) is temperature as well as heparin dependent. During bypass, as the patient's temperature decreases, the ACT increases unpredictably, but often to very high levels. Use of the ACT during hypothermic cardiopulmonary bypass as a criterion for administration of additional heparin is not at all valid. In practice there is seldom the necessity to administer more heparin during even two or three hours of cardiopulmonary bypass. There are now available heparin assays which can be useful at this stage to determine actual blood heparin level. The actual heparin levels remain remarkably constant during cardiopulmonary bypass. Little metabolic degradation occurs, probably due to hypothermia. There does not seem to be much need for additional heparin. This is a controversial statement, but it is based upon a large experience.

Protamine reversal of heparin after bypass is done in some centers again by calculating a dose response curve, but in other centers by a mg for mg substitution of protamine versus administration heparin dose. The new actual measurements of heparin levels will show whether or not there is residual heparin present after any method of reversal. It is reassuring to know whether or not there is free heparin present if patient is bleeding post bypass. There are also "protamine titration" methods for estimating remaining heparin level and thus calculating a sutiable dose of protamine. These methods have the common problem that the protamine titration method for measuring heparin level depends upon clotting and numerous other factors, and is thus inherently imprecise. We have not seen difficulties with the adminsitration of a reasonable overdose of protamine, and thus continue to calculate protamine dose based upon total administered heparin.

ARTERIAL PRESSURE ON BYPASS

This is another controversial subject. There are centers where "low flow, low pressure" bypass is utilized with apparently acceptable results with respect to neurologic damage post bypass. Early studies at Mayo Clinic indicated that reasonable oxygen delivery could be obtianed at pump flows of 2.0 to 2.4 $1/min/m^2$. These general guidelines are still followed in many centeres today. Arterial pressure is thought by many to be important during bypass because cerebral autoregulation permits normal cerebral blood flow at pressures down to, but not much below 50 mm Hg. Although high instances of neurologic damage have been reported following cardiopulmonary bypass in the past, and although these instances have been linked to arterial hypotension on bypass, there are other series which tend to refute this contention. A commonsense approach to this dilemma is to remember that, during hypothermia, oxygen demands are reduced dramatically. It is entirely possible that arterial pressure on bypass is not critically important during hypothermia, and becomes important only during rewarming. No one has proved this, but it seems prudent to become concerned about arterial pressure during this phase. During steady state hypothermic bypass at 25 to 29°C, we are not concerned if arterial pressure decreases to circa 30 mm Hg. In fact, permitting higher arterial pressures during the critical suturing of distal coronary anastomoses may result in excessive noncoronary collateral flow (despite aortic cross clamp). This may result in less than perfect surgical conditions and also may destroy the cardioplegia induced myocardial hypothermia; the most protective part of "cardioplegia". We see no reason to administer vasopressors during the hypothermic phase of cardiopulmonary bypass in an attempt to maintain some arbitrary pressure or other. On the other hand, during rewarming, we add phenylephrine or methoxamine to maintain arterial pressures at or above 50 mm Hg.

VASCULAR RESISTANCE OF BYPASS

Many feel that they cannot caluclate vascular resistance during bypass because they do not have an accurate measurement of the height of the venous reservoir level below the right atrium. In fact, the venous cannula in the right atrium constitutes a Starling resister Right atrial pressure can be taken as equal to atmospheric. Since this is true then: $\dfrac{MAP}{pump\ flow}$

WHAT ABOUT ADDING CO_2 DURING BYPASS?

This question has been controversial for years. If the Severinghaus correction factor is used to obtain an approximation of actual $PaCO_2$ during hypothermia, with no CO_2 added to the gas inflowing to the oxygenator, the actual $PaCO_2$'s will be disturbingly low. Thus, using temperature corrected blood gases will result in the addition of large amounts of CO_2, if any attempt is made to keep $PaCO_2$ in the 30 to 40 mm Hg range during bypass. If on the other hand, you are of the school of thought which says that blood gases during hypothermia should be drawn at whatever temperature, measured with 37°C electrodes, but not corrected back to actual perfusate temperature, then you will add less CO_2 during cardiopulmonary bypass. There are centers in fact wherein no CO_2 is added during cardiopulmonary bypass! The theorectical objection to such low $PaCO_2$'s is basically one of possible cerebral vasoconstriction. Human cerebral blood flow is probably not dramatically reduced at these low $PaCO_2$'s during cardiopulmonary bypass, relative to cerebral oxygen demands. Most perfuisonists, many of whom are caught in the middle of this dilemma, do add some CO_2 during cardiopulmonary bypass. They usually aim for "corrected" blood gases wherein the $PaCO_2$ is between 25 and 35 mm Hg. There are no hard outcome data which can refute or confirm this practice, but it does seem logical to take a "middle ground" stance between the two extremes mention above.

HYPERTENSION ON BYPASS

As time goes by, during hypothermic cardiopulmonary bypass, peripheral vascular resistance often inexorably increases, a fact which may result in excessive arterial pressure. "Breakthrough" of cerebral autoregulation may occur at or near mean arterial pressures of 150 mm Hg. It is possible that the patient is "protected" for cerebral hemorrhage below these pressures. Nonetheless, most anesthetists and perfusionists are unhappy with arterial pressures above 100 mm Hg on bypass based on clinical experience and many treat MAP > 70 mm Hg. The presence of such vasoconstriciton, in fact, is often seen an optimistic sign of vascular viability. The causes of such vasoconstriction have been variously attributed to catecholamine release, renin release, and generalized hypothermia. Whatever the cause, many anesthetists administer either nitroprusside or nitroglycerin during cardiopulmonary bypass. There is some preliminary evidence to indicate that perhaps nitroprusside-related cyanide toxicity might be <u>more</u> likely during hypothermic cardiopulmonary bypass than is usually the case. At SNP dosages of 5 ug/kg/min or less, Moore et al,* found excessive elevations of blood cyanide. They postulated that this might be due to continued <u>release</u> of cyanide (via nonenzymatic reaction with hemoglobin) during hypothermia, coupled with a relative failure of metabolic degradation of cyanide to thiocyanate, because of hypothermic depression of the liver enzyme rhodanese. Whatever the cause of this, nitroglycerin can be substituted during this phase of cardiopulmonary bypass. In addition to the above possible problem with nitroprusside, it has been shown to interfere with platelet aggregation. Once again, this may be something we don't need in pump cases. We would, for these several reasons, attempt to achieve vasodilation with nitroglycerin, rather than nitroprusside during cardiopulmonary bypass at least as a first line drug today. After the aortic crossclamp is removed, if there is any residual myocardial ischemia, we believe nitroglycerin to be the superior of the two vasodilators, because of its superior preload reduction effects.

LOW ARTERIAL PRESSURE GOING ON BYPASS

What do you do if there is near zero arterial pressure after the <u>perfusionist</u> announces reasonable flows just after going on bypass?
*Personal communication

108

The possibilities are several, all bad. It is possible that there is an aortic dissection occuring and that arterial inflow is into a different aortic lumen than that which is connected to the radial artery line. The dissection might also have occluded the subclavian artery, which is supplying your radial artery line. The absence of measureable arterial pressure during initial cardiopulmonary bypass warrants attention to the possibility of dissection. Another possibility, equally disastrous is that the circuit is set up backwards. Very low arterial pressures, circa 20 mm Hg are sometimes apparently due merely to decreased blood viscosity secondary to hemodilution. If there is some arterial pressure, then the above disasters are unlikely to have occurred. some have attributed this precipitous drop in arterial pressure on going on bypass to lack of pulsatile flow. This is illogical, because lack of pulsatility should be perceived by the baroreflexes as hypo, not hypertension and thus result in a sympathetic outpouring of vasoconstrictive impulses.

EMERGENCY BYPASS

The anesthetist should keep in mind that cardiopulmonary bypass can be used as an emergency measure. Critically ill or near-moribund patients can be placed on femoral vein femoral artery bypass under local anesthesia. When this is done, pump flows rarely exceed 2.0 l/min total. This is often sufficient to "rest" the failing heart and permit reasonable induction of anesthesia and commencement of surgery. For some reason, this relatively simple technique is often not considered as a help during induction of anesthesia in critically ill patients. The arterial inflow in this situation is via the femoral artery and, after sternotomy, the surgeon must obtain additional venous outflow via the right atrium, but this is seldom difficult.

RIGHT VENTRICULAR OUTFLOW RUPTURE

In some patients, almost always those who have had the privilege of cardiac surgery before, the heart will be stuck by adhesions to the underside of the sternum. If this is considered to be the case in advance, prudent cardiac surgeons will insert a femoral arterial line before incising the sternum. If right ventricular outflow tract disruption occurs during sternal splitting, and the femoral arterial cannula is in place, then the cardiotomy suction can be used to obtain some degree of venous return. Venous flow to the pump can be returned to the patient via the femoral cannula. It is important for the anesthetist to continue ventilation and all cardiac support as this kind of "bypass" is seldom adequate to supply total body needs. If right ventricular outflow tract rupture occurs in the absence of the above prudent precautions, then long periods of severe hypotension or circulatory arrest may result in neurologic damage.

CIRCULATORY ARREST ON BYPASS

Certain complex cngenital procedures such as the "takedown" of a Pott's anastomosis and other complex procedures require complete cessation of the circulation. For this, total body temperature is taken down to 12 to 17°C, at which point there is probably a period of 30 to 50 minutes during which safe circulatory arrest can be tolerated. It is critically important that the anesthetist administer a very large dose of neuromuscular blocker prior to circulatory arrest. During arrest, cerebral respiratory center pH/PCO2 will change in the direction to cause an intesne stimulation to diaphragmatic movement. The phrenic diaphragmatic myoneural junction is extremely difficult to completely block anyway. With this massive phrenic outpouring, it is possible for the diaphragm to begin movement during circulatory arrest. If a complex open cardiac procedure such as a Pott's takedown is occurring, it is possible to admit air to inaccessible places in the circulatory system. When bypass is resumed, said air may be propelled directly into the cerebral structures. Anesthetists not familiar with circulatory arrest have probably never experienced a time wherein appropriate therapeutic pharmacologic measures could not be undertaken. It is extremely frustrating, even scary, not to be able to administer any drugs.

AWARENESS DURING BYPASS

The point at which awareness is most likely is during rewarming. Cerebral structures are rewarmed rapidly because of relatively high blood flow. Volatile agents have probably been discontinued. Large doses of narcotics have likely been given previously, but are not total anesthetics in many patients. Thus we believe that early during the rewarming period is the time to administer some sort of hypnotic or amnesic agent. Lorazepam, 2 to 4 mg, diazepam 5 to 10 mg, or scopalomine 0.5 mg, can be given to accomplish this task. We do not see harm in routinely doing this, because it is difficult to decide whether or not awareness is occurring. During warming, profuse sweating is the rule rather than the exception. This does not mean awareness necessarily! It is important to remember that this sweating is most likely caused by hyperthermic hypothalamic perfusion. The hypothalamus is being perfused with blood of sufficient temperature to "convince" it to begin the sweating process. I have never noted the slightest correlation between awareness at this critical phase and sweating.

COMING OFF BYPASS

Many surgeons merely clamp the venous line and continue the pump flow at the previous high rate of speed, thus accomplishing a massive transfusion in short period of time. Physiologically, this amounts to placing an extreme hydraulic load in a very short period of time on a previously ischemic myocardium. This will almost always result in higher-than-necessary left ventricular preload. It is far better to gradually disconnect the patient from bypass with a slow transfusion, watching left atrial pressure or pulmonary capillary wedge pressure in the process. Some surgeons still believe that they can "feel" the left atrial pressure by placing their finger somewhere near the left atrium. Actually, the finger is resting on the right superior pulmonary vein, the pressure in which is equal to the left atrial pressure, but the wall thickness of which varies so greatly as to render this procedure essentially worthless. If your surgeon insists on coming off bypass by "feel" then I would insist on having a measurement of pulmonary capillary wedge pressure in order to come off bypass. If your surgeon insists on placing the now nearly outmoded left atrial line, then the use of the pulmonary capillary wedge pressure for this particular purpose is unnecessary. Left atrial lines require expert nursing care postoperatively to prevent inadvertant injection of air. Left atrial lines are constantly being "inadvertantly" removed by surgical assistants during the closure procedure. Left atrial lines are associated with bleeding and an occasional necessity to reoperate the patient in order to remove a recalcitrant line. All in all, I believe that surgeons should seldom find the need to insert a left atrial line. Complex congenital cardiac surgery is obviously an exception to the above statement.

HOW TO DECIDE ON AN INOTROPE

If a gradual and careful transfusion process has resulted in poor generation of pressure, i.e., systolic arterial pressure is less than 80 mm Hg, by the ventricle, in the face of increasing preload i.e., left atrial pressure is greater than 20 mm Hg or pulmonary capillary wedge pressure is greater than 25 mm Hg then we begin to consider the use of an inotrope. If it looks like minimal support will be needed, or first drug of choice would be dopamine, but we have a high index of suspicion for switching to the use of epinephrine, at this stage. It may well be prudent to add a vasodilator, usually nitroglycerin in our hands, early so as to produce reasonable left atrial pressures in response to the inotropic stimulus. If epinephrine and nitroglycerin have resulted in "fair" arterial pressures and cardiac indices in the "poor" to "fair" range, namely less than 1.8 $1/min/m^2$, we begin thinking about insertion of the intraortic balloon. We do not view the insertion of an intra-aortic balloon as a "defect" for our pharmacologic measures. The balloon is the only sure way to separate myocardial oxygen supply from demand. During routine cardiopulmonary bypass procedures for coronary artery disease, the balloon should seldom be necessary, but if your practice includes severely ill patients with valvular disease or combinations of coronary artery and valvular disease, the above comments will be appreciated.

PULSATILE VERSUS NON PULSATILE BYPASS

Over the years, many attempts have been made to reproduce normal cardiovascular pulsatility during bypass. These devices are always more complex than the simple roller pumps inow in widespread use. Various advantages of pulsatile bypass have been claimed over the years. Nonetheless, non pulsatile bypass have proven itself in many hundreds of cases and, because is probably cheaper and certainly simpler, it will likely remain in widespread use until major and definitive outcome-related advantages are shown for pulsatile flow during cardiopulmonary bypass.

SUGGESTED READING

1. Ionescu MI, Wooler GH: Current techniques in extra corporeal circulation. Butterworths, London 1976.
2. Kaplan JA: Cardiac Anesthesia. Grune & Stratton, New York 1979.
3. Ball MH, Huse WM, Bull BS: Evaluation of tests used to monitor heparin therapy during extracorporeal circulation. Anesthesiology 1975;43:346.
4. Stockard JJ, Bickford RG, Schauble JF: Pressure dependent cerebral ischemia during cardiopulmonary bypass. J Neurol 1973;23:521.
5. Messmer K, Schmid-Schonobein H: Hemodilution: Theoretical basis and clinical application. Adv Cardiol, Basel, Karger, 1972.

CEREBRAL BLOOD FLOW DURING BYPASS (IS PRESSURE IMPORTANT?)

ANN V. GOVIER, M.D., ROBERT D. MCKAY, M.D., J.G. REVES, M.D.

Introduction

The incidence of transient post cardiac surgery neurologic dysfunction varies between 0 and 40%.[1-14] Slogoff has shown that this incidence depends on the retrospective vs. prospective and sensitivity vs. specificity of the studies.[14] (Table). Hypotension has been implicated as a precipitating cause by a number of investigators[2,3,5,6,11] while others have failed to show a correlation of hypotension with cerebral dysfunction.[8,14] We wished to examine the relationship of cerebral blood flow and perfusion pressure during cardio-pulmonary bypass (CPB). If cerebral autoregulation is lost during CPB, it is possible that hypotension could produce decreased cerebral perfusion. The

STUDIES REPORTING INCIDENCE OF CEREBRAL DYSFUNCTION AFTER OPEN HEART OPERATIONS

Year (Ref.)	No. of Patients	P/R	C/P	Incidence Transient	Persistent	I/E	Prime
1961 (1)	244	R	C	7.0	1.6	I	NR
1965 (2)	35	P	C&P	34.0	23.0	I	NR
1965 (9)	78	P	C&P	38.0	NR	I	NR
1967 (10)	53	P	C&P	13.0	13.0	I	NR
1970 (3)	85	P	C&P	44.0	15.0	I	B
1971 (11)	71	P	C&P	31.0	NR	I	B
1972 (12)	417	R	C	19.2	9.1	I	B
1973 (5)	25	P	C	36.0	12.1	I&E	NR
1975 (6)	528	R	C	7.4	4.8	I&E	B
1977 (4)	223	P	C&P	8.5	NR	I&E	B&C
1980 (7)	30	P	C&P	O	O	E	C
1980 (13)	418	R	C	16.0	NR	E	NR
1980 (8)	204	P	C&P	40.0	17.2	I&E	C
1980 (15)	170	R	C	NR	5.3	E	C
1982 (14)	204	P	C&P	16.2	6.4	I&E	C

Abbreviations used are: P/R = perspective: P = prospective,R = retrospective; C/P = type of observation: C = clinical, P = psychometric; I/E = closed or open operation: I = intracardiac, E = extracardiac; B = blood; C = crystalloid only; NR = not reported. (retyped from reference #14).

reduced perfusion could then produce central nervous system (CNS) hypoxia and contribute to CNS damage if the oxygen delivery were insufficient to meet oxygen demand. We used a method of cerebral blood flow determination during CPB first reported by McKay et al.[16] and recently used by Henriksen et al.[17]

Methods

After Institutional Review Board approval for human study, regional cerebral blood flow (rCBF) was determined by ^{133}Xe clearance[18] in 14 patients undergoing coronary artery bypass graft surgery anesthetized with diazepam 0.3–0.5 mg/kg, fentanyl 10–20 mcg/kg and N_2O/O_2 50:50. Patients with known cerebrovascular disease or with hypertension (diastolic BP $\geq$ 90 mmHg) were excluded. CBF was determined by injecting saline containing 300 µCi of ^{133}Xe into the left common carotid artery and obtaining clearance curves from a single extracranial scintillation detector placed perpendicular to the scalp approximately over the left Rolandic fissure (Fig. 1). The rCBF was measured during CPB at different mean arterial blood pressures but at a constant pump flow of 1.6 L/min/m[2], $PaCO_2$ of 32–38 mmHg (temperature uncorrected) and nasopharyngeal temperature of 25–30° C. Mean rCBF values were compared by analysis of variance and linear regression analysis was performed to determine correlation coefficients between rCBF and blood pressure and hemoglobin. Neurologic tests were not performed before or after surgery.

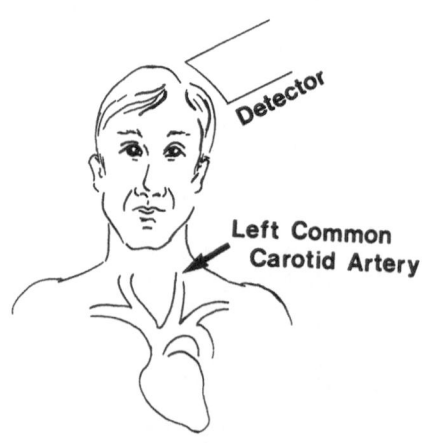

FIGURE 1.

Results

Twenty-five observations were made in 14 patients. The mean $PaCO_2$ was 35 ± 2.2 mmHg, pump flow 1.6 ± 0.00 L/min/m^2 and temperature $28 \pm 1.2^\circ$ C. MAP ranged from 30 to 113 mmHg, rCBF ranged from 7.8 to 15.6 ml/100g/min and Hb ranged from 5.6 to 11.1 g/dl. The association of rCBF and MAP (Fig. 2) was relatively poor ($r = .44$, $p < .03$). There was a relatively good association of rCBF with Hb ($r = -.63$, $p < .001$, Fig. 3) and of MAP with Hb ($r = .62$, $p < .001$). No patients developed any grossly apparent neurologic dysfunction in the postoperative period.

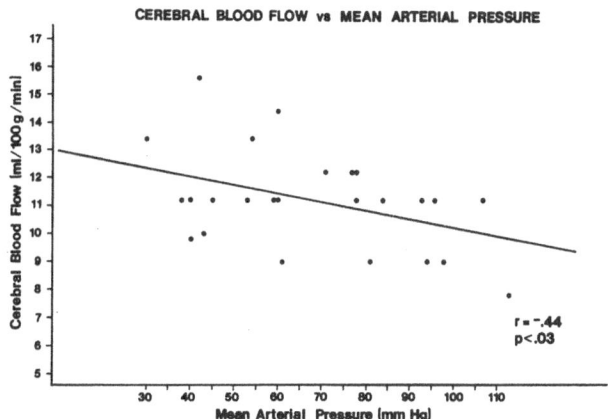

FIGURE 2.

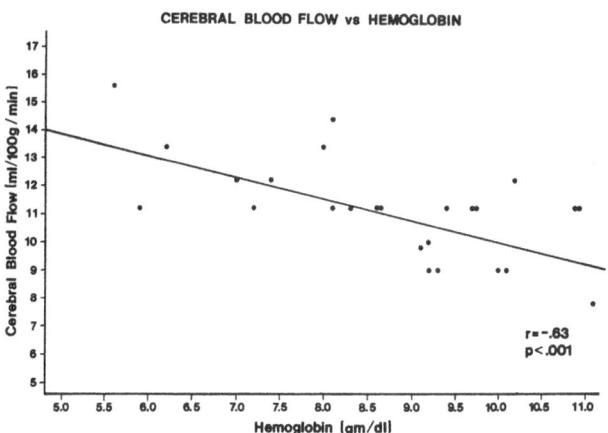

FIGURE 3.

Discussion

In normotensive humans at normothermia and with normal cerebrovascular status, autoregulation allows the cerebral circulation to maintain constant CBF between a MAP of 50 to 150 mmHg. We found a poor association of rCBF and MAP during CPB which is consistent with preserved metabolic regulation during CPB in moderately hypothermic patients. In fact, CPB appears to extend the lower limit of autoregulation to at least 30 mmHg. The inverse relationship between rCBF and Hb may indicate that hemodilution improves rCBF during CPB and/or that adequate oxygen delivery is maintained by autoregulation. Patients in this study were not exposed to hypercarbia and did not receive volatile anesthetic agents - both of which may impair cerebral autoregulation.

The data from our study[19] indicate that pharmacologic treatment of arterial pressures between 30 and 110 mmHg is not necessary to insure a constant cerebral blood flow. There is no evidence from this study to indicate that a MAP less than 50 mmHg is accompanied by a decrease in rCBF. Since we did not correlate the changes in rCBF with postoperative neurologic function, we cannot establish a relationship of rCBF with postoperative CNS function. However, the recommendation to maintain a perfusion pressure $\geq$ 50 mmHg during CPB[5] cannot be defended solely on the premise that increased MAP will increase rCBF. It appears that factors other than the level of arterial pressure are important in determining cerebral blood flow during CPB. One such factor probably is temperature; the reduction in rCBF during CPB is likely related to the calculated 40% reduction in cerebral metabolic rate for O_2 ($CMRO_2$) expected with the 8° C decrease in temperature, assuming the Q10 for human brain to be 2.0.[20] If the relationship between metabolism and flow remains coupled, as the metabolic requirement decreases, so will the flow. Additional studies are necessary to determine whether there is a critical level of blood pressure below which cerebral blood flow can become inadequate, causing disorders of cerebral function to occur.

Our rCBF data are at variance with that reported by the Copenhagen group.[17] They found an increase in rCBF during CPB in moderately hypothermic patients (from 38 ml/100g/min to 64 ml/100g/min, p < .01). It is difficult to explain this surprising discrepancy in the data since the methodology was almost identical. They postulated that the increase in rCBF that they found might be due to "uncoupling of flow and metabolism" perhaps due to microvascular blockade by emboli or the non-physiologic conditions of CPB (hemodilution, non-pulsatile flow, changes in ^{133}Xe blood-tissue partition coefficients). The "luxury perfusion" they report is difficult to understand. They also found that cerebral autoregulation was lost at perfusion pressures below 55 mmHg. Below this level, CBF was significantly correlated with perfusion pressure (p < 0.01).[17] This data is also at variance with our data in which we found preservation of autoregulation down to 30 mmHg during CPB. Their patients did receive volatile anesthetics which are known to impair cerebral autoregulation.[21,22]

Summary

In conclusion, it appears that during CPB at flows of 1.6 L/min/m^2 in moderately hypothermic patients, the lower limit of autoregulation is extended, and that pharmacologic support is not necessary to maintain a constant cerebral blood flow between a MAP of 30 to 110 mmHg. It is not known whether the low rCBF encountered during CPB contributes to subclinical neurologic dysfunction. Investigations are planned to explore this question.

References

1. Ehrenhaft JL, Claman MA, Layton Jm, Zimmerman GR: Cerebral complications of open heart surgery; further observations. J Thorac Cardiovasc Surg 42:514-526, 1961
2. Gilman S: Cerebral disorders after open-heart operations. N Engl J Med 272:489-498, 1965
3. Tufo HM, Ostfeld AM, Shekelle R: Central nervous system dysfunction following open-heart surgery. JAMA 212:1333-1340, 1970
4. Aberg T, Kihlgren M: Cerebral protection during open-heart surgery. Thorax 32:525-533, 1977
5. Stockard JJ, Bickford RG, Schauble JF: Pressure dependent cerebral ischemia during cardiopulmonary bypass. Neurology 23:521-529, 1973
6. Branthwaite MA: Prevention of neurological damage during open-heart surgery. Thorax 30:258-261, 1975
7. Ellis RJ, Wisniewski A, Potts R, Calhoun C, Loucks P, Wells MR: Reduction of flow rate and arterial pressure at moderate hypothermia does not result in cerebral dysfunction. J Thorac Cardiovasc Surg 79:173-180, 1980
8. Kolkka R, Hilberman M: Neurologic dysfunction following cardiac operation with low flow, low pressure cardiopulmonary bypass. J Thorac Cardiovasc Surg 79:432-437, 1980
9. Kornfeld DS, Zimberg S, Malm JR: Psychiatric complications of open-heart surgery. N Engl J Med 273:287-292, 1965
10. Gilbertstadt H, Sako Y: Intellectual and personality changes following open-heart surgery. Arch Gen Psychiatry 16:210-214, 1967
11. Lee WH, Brady MP, Rowe JM, Miller WC Jr: Effects of extracorporeal circulation upon behavior, personality and brain function. II. Hemodynamic metabolic and psychometric correlations. Ann Surg 173:1013-1023, 1971
12. Branthwaite MA: Neurologic damage related to open-heart surgery. Thorax 27:748-753, 1972

13. Breuer AC, Furlan AJ, Hanson MR, et al: Neurologic complications of open-heart surgery: computer associated analysis of 531 patients. Cleve Clin Q 48:205-206, 1981

14. Slogoff S, Girgis KZ, Keats AS: Etiologic factors in neuropsychiatric complications associated with cardiopulmonary bypass. Anesth Analg 61:903-911, 1982

15. Turnipseed WD, Berkoff HA, Belzer FO: Postoperative stroke in cardiac and peripheral vascular disease. Ann Surg 192:365-368, 1980

16. McKay RD, Reves JG, Karp RB, Morawetz RB, Lell WA: Effects of cardiopulmonary bypass on cerebral blood flow. Anesth Analg 62:274-275, 1983

17. Henriksen L, Hjelms E, Lindeburgh T: Brain hyperfusion during cardiac operations. Thoracic (in press)

18. Waltz AG, Wanek AR, Anderson RE: Comparison of analytic methods for calculation of cerebral blood flow after intracarotid injection of ^{133}Xe. J Nucl Med 13:66-72, 1972

19. Govier AV, Reves JG, McKay RD, et al: Relationship of cerebral blood flow and perfusion pressure during cardiopulmonary bypass. (Abstract) Anesthesiology (in press)

20. Siesjo BK: Brain Energy Metabolism. New York: John Wiley and Sons, 1978, p 331

21. Morita H, Bleyaert AL, Stezoski SW, Stezoski SW, Nemoto EM: The effect of halothane anesthesia on cerebral blood flow, autoregulation and cerebral metabolism of oxygen and glucose. Abstracts of Scientific Papers, ASA Annual Meeting, 1974, pp 63-64

22. Murphy FL, Kennell EM, Johnstone RE, et al: The effects of enflurane, isoflurane, and halothane on cerebral blood flow and metabolism in man. Abstracts of Scientific Papers, ASA Annual Meeting, 1974, pp 61-62

HYPERTENSION DURING AND AFTER CARDIOPULMONARY BYPASS

F. G. ESTAFANOUS, M.D.

The BP is only one aspect in a highly integrated cardiovascular system. It is controlled by many variables: cardiac output, peripheral resistance and blood volume, which are in turn controlled by autonomic centers, mechanical factors, hormones and neurogenic reflexes.[1] Surgery anesthesia, and cardiopulmonary bypass effect all these variables, and it is not surprising if either hypertension or hypotension occur during cardiovascular surgery or in the postoperative period.

Hypertension related to surgery was first recognized in 1902 when Cushing[2] was the first to detect serious postoperative hypertension due to increased intracranial tension following brain surgery. Later, hypertension due to postnatal eclampsia was recognized and managed. By 1957,[3] deaths were reported due to hypertension following resection for thoracic aortic coarctation.

In 1972 we first described a high incidence of severe, transient systemic hypertension complicating myocardial revascularization in 35%[4] of patients and in 5-10% of patients[5] following heart valve replacement, and a much higher incidence following aortic and carotid surgery. Since then we realized more that hypertension is a definite complication during and after major cardiovascular surgery.

Definition of Hypertension:

A rise in BP does not mean hypertension by definition. In all our studies we restricted the term "hypertension" to the situation where the rise in BP can cause complications and does require treatment. In preoperatively normotensives (BP < 140/90 mmHg), a rise in BP of up to 160 systolic or 100 diastolic is considered to be a hypertensive episode. As preoperative hypertensives (BP > 160/100) are more prone to a rise in BP, a rise in either systolic or diastolic pressure of 20 mmHg above the preoperative value usually requires treatment. The rise in BP can be due to general sympathetic stimulation as well as to specific, mechanical, hormonal or neural factors.

General Causes of Hypertension in a Surgical and Postoperative Set-up
Postoperative Hypoxia and Hypercarbia:

In their early stages, postoperative hypoxia and hypercarbia cause a gradual increase in both the heart rate and BP. If untreated, the rise in BP continues and can be severe until the vasomotor center fails. Thereafter bradycardia and hypotension engender a situation which may be irreversible. In a postsurgical set up, variable degrees of hypoxia and/or hypercarbia are expected due to the residual effects of pain medications, anesthetics, muscle relaxants, and due to the interference of the surgical incision and procedure involving the respiratory muscles. Even in a mechanically ventilated patient, hypoxia or hypercarbia cannot be excluded due to mechanical failure of ventilators, disconnection of tubing and tension pneumothorax.[6]

If unexplained hypertension occurs, it is important to rule out hypoxia, hypercarbia and pain as causes of this rise in BP and to treat them specifically before initiation of any peripheral vasodilatory therapy. The use of peripheral vasodilators to treat hypertension caused by hypoxia and hypercarbia will cause a serious and profound drop in BP, as it counteracts the compensatory vasoconstriction.

Preoperatively hypertensive patients are expected to have a more pronounced rise in BP in response to sympathetic factors.[7] However, results of our studies of more than 200 hypertensive patients for whom antihypertensive therapy was continued until the time of surgery, revealed that the incidence of POH, according to the levels we properly defined, was not any higher than the incidence in preoperatively normotensive patients.[4]

BP Changed During Cardiopulmonary Bypass:

On initiation of cardiopulmonary bypass, arterial mean pressure usually drops by as much as 40-50%, but it begins rising toward pre-bypass values within a few minutes.[8] The fall and subsequent rise in arterial pressure are not related to changes in cardiac output since these develop while the aorta is cross-clamped and the heart is excluded from the circulation. Also, the changes in mean arterial pressure do not always reflect the changes that occur in the pump output; the rise in arterial pressure is therefore very much related to variations in peripheral vascular resistance. The cause and mechanism(s) for these variations have not been fully elucidated. Factors mentioned include dilutions of priming solutions, histamine release, increased ADH and alterations of circulating catecholamines.[9,10] As concerns the latter, most reports to-date have been analyzed in unifactorial terms rather than as part of a complex of interacting mechanisms.[11] In a situation entailing cross-clamping and manipulation of the aorta, activation of reflex pressor mechanisms[12] could be postulated. Less speculative are changes in circulating angiotensin(AII) levels consequent to cardiopulmonary bypass.

Taylor et al[13] have shown that plasma AII levels were markedly higher during nonpulsatile bypass and that this increase could be attenuated by using pulsatile flow. Alterations in peripheral vascular resistance were said to correlate closely with changes in plasma AII; further arterial pressure and vascular resistance fell significantly following the infusions of captopril.[13] The evidence appears quite impressive but it was derived only from observations or experiments in which mean arterial pressure was not increased. The extension of these conclusions to hypertension was only inferential; despite the high levels of plasma AII reported, no actual hypertensive episode was described. That nonpulsatile flow can activate the renin angiotensin system, and that increased AII can lead to marked vasoconstriction both appear plausible; their casual relationship to intraoperative hypertension has not yet been demonstrated directly. Hypertensive episodes during cardiopulmonary bypass have not been infrequent in our experience; Roberts et al[14] did not mention any in their series of 100 consecutive operations. However, when the BP rises during bypass it usually does not respond either to deepening the level of anesthesia or to reducing pump flow, but it is usually controlled by vasodilators. In all of our previous studies of postoperative hypertension, this rise of blood pressure was not correlated with the subsequent development of hypertension in the postoperative period.

Hemodynamic Alterations Following Cardiopulmonary Bypass:

The hemodynamic changes that follow cardiopulmonary bypass usually follow a uniform and rather interesting pattern. These changes can explain in part or all why post-bypass hypertension is a major complication of cardiac surgery.

Our studies in patients with good ventricular function[15] undergoing coronary artery surgery demonstrated that the pattern of hemodynamic changes following cardiopulmonary bypass consist of: immediate decrease in SVR and increase in CO when the right and left ventricular filling pressures were maintained at preoperative levels by transfusion. The drop in SVR can be ascribed to hemodilution. Previous hemodynamic studies, both experimental and clinical, confirmed that cardiac output will increase markedly in patients with good ventricular function in response to reduction in the circulating red cell mass[16] confirming what Guyton and Richardson demonstrated in 1960.[17]

In our studies, the increased output compensated fully for the reduced SVR and the patients did not become hypotensive, however, late in surgery and early postoperatively the SVR began to rise and continued to do so despite the presence of hemodilution. Concomitantly, the elevated CO began to decrease returning to the initial preoperative values. The MAP usually rises significantly to higher levels than immediately post-bypass and can reach levels higher than those measured in the initial control period and also can reach the levels we defined as hypertensive episodes. The systemic vascular resistance usually increases significantly from the post-bypass value. This is remarkable because of the persistence of hemodilution and the presumed low viscosity.

This hemodynamic pattern of increasing SVR and BP with practically unchanged levels of CO in the presence of unchanged pulmonary capillary wedge pressure and central venous pressure, resembles the hemodynamic pattern of postmyocardial revascularization hypertension that we initially described.[4] At this point it is worth re-emphasizing that these studies were performed in patients with good ventricular function. These patients were capable of increasing their cardiac output and maintaining their BP in the presence of hemodilution. Also, when the SVR increased, the cardiac output was maintained close to the control values without significant change in the filling pressures and without ventricular distention. However, in patients with left ventricular impairment, the diseased myocardium imposes strict limits on the volume of blood that can be ejected by the heart, despite the needs and status of the peripheral circulation.[18] The weakened heart may not have the same response to the increased preload. In this situation, hypotension may be inevitable, when the SVR increases significantly increasing the afterload, the response of the impaired heart may be also different, as further increase in the afterload can impose limitations on the cardiac output. In this situation, a decreased cardiac output may limit the rise of blood pressure and the incidence of hypertension. Cardiogenic reflexes have been implicated in the genesis of the rise in SVR and this hypertension;[19] their exact role still remains to be determined precisely.

Throughout all our studies of hemodynamic alterations during cardiac surgery, the hematocrit level correlated significantly with CO, however, arterial pressures did not correlate with the changes in CO. Arterial pressure variations correlated strongly with SVR signifying that pressure was mainly dependent on changes in vascular resistance.[16] Although SVR is a calculated value dependent on some theoretical assumptions, its variations in short-term situations can be considered as a clinically valid index of changes in vascular caliber.[20]

We could not demonstrate that hormonal changes were a factor in the genesis of these characteristic hemodynamic patterns. Plasma renin activity did not change significantly; neither did serum norepinephrine or serum epinephrine. Continuation of preoperative beta adrenergic blockers until the time of surgery may have obtunded the humoral responses[21] reported by others.[22] Whatever the case, we found no significant correlation between changes in SVR and variations in either plasma renin activity, serum epinephrine, or serum norepinephrine levels. We concluded from our studies that:

a) In this clinical setting, the changes in SVR were more important in determining MAP levels than changes in CO.

b) Patients with good ventricular function who are capable of increasing their CO in response to hemodilution and decreased SVR vary from patients with impaired ventricular function who might not be able to increase their CO or to adjust their filling pressures to increases in SVR.

Hypertension Following Cardiovascular Surgery:

General Causes: Paroxysmal hypertension in the immediate post-bypass period is a frequent and potentially dangerous condition. The precipitating factors could be many: arousal from anesthesia, tracheal and nasopharyngeal manipulations, pain, hypothermia, shivering, poor ventilation and the use of pressor agents as well as the wearing off of antihypertensive medications. In addition, postoperative coronary insufficiency or myocardial infarct might also raise blood pressure; signs of cardioadrenergic stimulation were particularly marked following coronary bypass in those patients who sustained a postoperative infarction.[23] Hypervolemia is often cited as a possible cause of postoperative hypertension. The relationship of fluid overload to increased arterial pressure is, however, more complex than a relationship of container and content.[24] Compensatory neural mechanisms can adequately buffer sizeable blood volume variations;[25] only in the functional absence of such reflexes or of renal excretory function with arterial pressure correlate directly with hypervolemia.[26] On the other hand, marked sympathetic reaction to hypovolemia could be an unrecognized cause of serious hypertension and impaired tissue perfusion.[27]

Hyertension Following Surgery on the Thoracic Aorta:

Resection of thoracic aortic coarctation complicated by two types of POH was reported as early as 1957.[3] Early hypertension occurs either during or immediately after surgery. It is usually benign, lasts for a few hours, and responds to treatment. In our experience, the hemodynamic characteristics of this immediate type of hypertension are rather similar to those of post myocardial revascularization that are described later. This type of delayed hypertension is easily controlled by peripheral vasodilators. Practically speaking, it is almost always prevented by the use of vasodilators with the initial signs of a rise in BP. However, previously this type of hypertension almost passed unnoticed but more attention was paid to the immediate type of hypertension which was complicated by a high incidence of mortality and morbidity.

Delayed hypertension occurs in more than 20% of patients.[28] The BP usually starts to rise 24 to 48 hours postoperatively. Deceivingly, the rise in BP is usually manifested by severe intra-abdominal pain, resembling acute appendicitis or acute abdomen due to accompanying mesenteric endarteritis. Following resection of aortic coarctation, the pressure proximal to the coarctation decreases the baroreceptors which were adjusted to the high pressure and reduces their inhibitor impulses to the vasomotor centers. The sympathetic activity and circulating catecholamines increase, causing severe vasoconstriction and hypertension. This unexpected rise in catecholamine levels will cause severe spasm of the mesenteric vessels and mesenteric thrombosis and gangrene. Again, control of the BP at the early stages of this hypertension almost eliminated these complications.

Hypertension Following Valve Replacement:

The results of our studies of 185 patients who had cardiac valve replacement showed that up to as many as 10% of patients are hypertensive after aortic valve replacement as are 5% of patients who had mitral valve replacement.[5] The rise in BP usually starts a few hours post-operatively, and it is not related to preoperative lesions, hypervolemia, use of hypothermia during surgery, or to the type of prosthesis used. The cause of such rise in BP can be partially attributed to improvement in the hemodynamics following valve replacement or to stimulation of afferent pressor reflexes from the heart, a mechanism similar to that of hypertension which follows coronary artery surgery, since the hemodynamic patterns is similar.

Postmyocardial Revascularization Hypertension:

Since our original description of post-myocardial revascularization hypertension in 1973, it became recognized as possibly the most common complication of coronary bypass surgery.[4] It occurs in 30-50% of patients; much higher than the incidence following cardiac valve replacement (5-10%). This difference can be attributed to the instability of blood pressure control, reduced baroreceptor sensitivity, and the frequent hypovolemia in patients with coronary artery disease.[29] Most investigators have outlined the following clinical syndrome with typical hemodynamic characteristics. The increase in arterial pressure occurs during the first four hours after operation. The BP increases gradually, but steadily, despite sedation and well controlled ventilation. The increase in pressure can be severe and exceeds systolic pressure by 60 mmHg or more. Despite the increase in pressure, there is no slowing of the heart rate: on the contrary, it can be slightly higher with occasional premature ventricular complexes.[4] The central venous and the left atrial pressures remain within normal limits. A search for predisposing factors by our group and other investigators did not produce any consistent results. Most authors agree that the type of anesthetic agents used, the duration of cardiopulmonary bypass, and the distribution of coronary artery lesions did not significantly influence the incidence of postoperative hypertension. Our impression was that this hypertension occurred more frequently among patients with well preserved myocardial function.

In all published reports, the increase in BP after coronary bypass surgery was related to a significant increase in total peripheral resistance.[30] The change in hemodynamic pattern as pressure increased was the same in all patients with no significant change in either cardiac output or central venous or left atrial pressures. Indeed, these findings helped us to discount hypervolemia as a cause for this hypertension. There were two paradoxical findings associated with the increase in pressure: 1) lack of slowing of the heart rate and 2) further elevations of the mean rate of left ventricular ejection. This hemodynamic pattern suggested an increased sympathetic drive that in turn, helped to explain why cardiac output was not reduced.

Several authors reported a correlation between the increased arterial pressure and elevation in plasma catecholamine levels.[31] There is a possible role for the activities of the renin/angiotensin system which is reported in some cases.[32] As these correlations are not very close, this suggests the possible role of a reflex mechanism. The success of stellate ganglion blockade in lowering the total peripheral resistance and consequently controlling the hypertension speaks in favor of a reflex mechanism.

As early as 1973 we postulated that the sympathetic overdrive was possibly related to the activation of pressor reflexes from the heart, great vessels or coronary arteries. Similar pressor reflexes originating from the coronary arteries, the heart, and the great vessels were described by Malliani, Brown, and James.[33,34] The previous work of Tarazi et al[35] demonstrated that stellate ganglion stimulation can produce hypertension as well as the lack of any previous predilection of post coronary bypass hypertension for operations on any single coronary bed. This suggested that of the various possible pressor reflexes, the more important in this contest were those that involved sympathetic afferent fibers.

We therefore elected to test the effect of unilateral stellate ganglion block in patients with hypertension after coronary bypass surgery. Both in our initial series and in a subsequent larger group of patients, an effective unilateral block resulted in rapid and definitive normalization of arterial pressure in the vast majority of cases.[36] The reduction in BP was rapid, smooth and related to a decrease in SVR with no evidence of diminished cardiac performance. These results were interpreted to indicate that the BP response was probably due to our interrruption of afferent fibers coursing through or relaying in either stellate ganglion.

The success of stellate block does not mean that all causes of hypertension after coronary bypass surgery are due to pressor reflexes from the sympathetic afferent fibers. A possible role for an activated angiotension system cannot be ignored. However, even if this is confirmed, it does not necessarily contradict a cardiac origin of this hypertension, because sympathetic stimulation is an important cause of renin release.

Whatever the causes and timing of hypertension, it is a serious complication for patients recovering from open heart surgery. The increase in pressure and in total peripheral resistance increases cardiac work and myocardial oxygen consumption. Previous studies demonstrated that the endocardial viability ratio as well as the ratio of diastolic to systolic pressure time indexes were lower in patients who had postoperative hypertension than in those who remained normotensive.[37,38] The decrease in these indexes means an increased susceptability to subendocardial ischemia which can be further aggravated by the anemia due to the hemodilution that is often used in heart surgery.

Hypertension also increases the risk of cerebral vascular accidents. The incidence and amount of postoperative bleeding in a previously heparinized patient are much greater during hypertension.

Therefore, it is evident that every effort should be made to prevent, control, and to treat hypertension promptly and adequately during various stages of heart surgery.

Treatment:

Unilateral stellate ganglion blockade was effective in our experience for rapid normalization of the elevated BP in a large number of patients who developed hypertension after myocardial revascularization. It was also effective in those with hypertensive episodes immediately after heart valve replacement. We have even found stellate block to be effective when large doses of peripheral vasodilators failed to adequately control the paroxysmal increase in pressure. However, unless this blockade is performed with great care, by a physician trained in its use, the incidence of its success rate can be quite low. More importantly, it can be complicated by pneumothorax, hemothorax or nerve injury. Bilateral stellate block is dangerous because of the possibility of undue cardiac depression.

Sodium nitroprusside is the most consistently effective drug of choice for hypertension associated with acute coronary insufficiency and left ventricular impairment. We use it routinely for treatment of post myocardial revascularization and we only resort to stellate blockade on rare occasions when large amounts of sodium nitroprusside are required or when it fails to control the blood pressure.

REFERENCES

1. Froelich ED, Tarazi RC, Dustan HP: Re-examination of the hemodynamics of hypertension. Am J Med Sci 275:9-23, 1969.
2. Cushing: Journal of Medical Sciences, September, 1902.
3. Groves LK, Effler DB: Problems in surgical management of coarctation of the aorta. J Thorac Cardiovaasc Surg 19:60-90, 1960.
4. Estafanous FG, Tarazi RC, Viljoen JF, et al: Systemic hypertension following myocardial revascularization. Am Heart J 85:732-8, 2973
5. Estafanous FG, Tarazi RC, Buckley S, et al: Arterial hypertension in immediate postoperative period after valve replacement. Br Heart J 40:718-24, 1978.
6. Estafanous FG, Viljoen JF, Barsoum KN: Diagnosis of pneumothorax complicating mechanical ventilation. Anes Analg 54:730-735, 1975.
7. Prys-Roberts C, Greene LT, Meloche R, Foex P: Studies of anesthesia in relation to hypertension. II. Haemodynamic consequences of induction and endotracheal intubation. Br J Anaesth 43:531-46, 1971.
8. Tan CK, Glisson SN, El-Etr AA, Ramakrishnaiah KB: Levels of circulating norepinephrine and epinephrine before, during and after cardiopulmonary bypass in man. J Thorac Cardiovasc Surg 71:928-32, 1976.
9. Anton AH, Gravenstein JS, Wheat MW: Extracorporeal circulation and endogenous epinephrine and norepinephrine in plasma, atrium and urine in man. Anesthesiology 25:262-9, 1964.

10. Hine IP, Wood WG, Mainwaring-Burton RW, Butler MJ, Irving MH, Booker B: The adrenergic response to surgery involving cardiopulmonary bypass, as measured by plasma and urinary catecholamine concentrations. Br J Anaesth 48:355-62, 1976.
11. Tarazi RC, Gifford RW: Systemic arterial pressure. In:Sodeman WA Jr, Sodeman TM eds. Pathophysiology. Philadelphia:WB Saunders:198-229, 1979.
12. Malliani A, Peterson DF, Biship VS, Brown AM: Spinal sympathetic cardiovascular reflexes. Circ Res 30:158-66, 1972.
13. Taylor KM, Brannan JJ, Bain WH, Caves PK, Morton IJ: Vasoconstriction during cardiopulmonary bypass. Cardiovasc Res 13:269-73, 1979.
14. Roberts AJ, Niarchos AP, Subramanian VA et al: Systemic hypertension associated with coronary artery bypass surgery. J Thorac Cardiovasc Surg 74:846-59, 1977.
15. Urzua J, Estafanous FG, Tarazi RC, et al: Cardiac performance following cardiopulmonary bypass. Presented at the Society of Cardiovascular Anesthesiologists 3rd Annual Meeting, San Francisco, May, 1981.
16. Estafanous FG, Urzua J, Yared JP, Zurick AM, Loop FD, Tarazi RC: Pattern of hemodynamic alterations during coronary artery surgery. Accepted for publication in J Thorac Cardiovasc Surg.
17. Guyton AC, Richardson TQ: Effect of hematocrit on venous return. Circ Res 9:157-64, 1961.
18. Peterson DF, Brown AM: Pressor reflexes produced by stimulation of afferent fibers in the cardiac sympathetic nerves of the cat. Circ Res 28:605-10, 1971.
19. Fouad FM, Estafanous FG, Tarazi RC: Post coronary bypass hypertension: Evidence of its reflex origin. Circulation 55 & 56 (supplement 3):III-30, 1977.
20. Tarazi RC, Gifford RW Jr: Systemic arterial pressure. In: Pathologic Physiology. Edited by Sodeman WA, Sodeman WA Jr, Philadelphia, WB Saunders, 5th ed, 1974, pp:177-205.
21. Myers JH, Horwitz LD: Hemodynamic and metabolic response after abrupt withdrawal of long-term propranolol. Circulation 58:196-201, 1978.
22. Taylor KM, Morton IJ, Brown JJ, et al: Hypertension and the renin-angiotensin system following open heart surgery. J Thorac Cardiovasc Surg 74:840-5, 1977.
23. Boudoulas H, Lewis RP, Vasko JS, et al: Left ventricular function and adrenergic hyperactivity before and after saphenous vein bypass. Circulation 53:802-6, 1976.
24. Tarazi RC: Hemodynamic role of extracellular fluid in hypertension. Circ Res 38:Suppl II:ii-72-83, 1976.
25. Leutscher JA, Boyers DG, Cuthbertson JF, McMahon DF: A model of the human circulation. Circ Res 32 & 33: Suppl I:I-84-98.
26. Dustan HP, Tarazi RC, Braco EL, Dart RA: Plasma and extracellular fluid volumes in hypertension. Circ Res 32 & 33: Suppl I:I-73-83.
27. Cohn JN: Paroxysmal hypertension and hypovolemia. N Engl J Med 275:643-6, 1966.
28. Sealy WC: Coarction of the aorta and hypertension. Ann Thorac Surg 3:15-28, 1967.
29. Estafanous FG, Tarazi RC: Systemic arterial hypertension associated with cardiac surgery. Am J Cardiol 46:685-94, 1980.

30. Fouad FM, Estafanous FG, Tarazi RC: Hemodynamics of postmyocardial revascularization hypertension. Am J Cardiol 41:564-9, 1978.
31. Fouad FM, Estafanous FG, Bravo EL, Iyer KA, Maydak JH, Tarazi RC: Possible role of cardio-aortic reflexes in postcoronary bypass hypertension. Am J Cardiol 44:866-72, 1976.
32. Niarchos AP, Roberts AJ, Case DB, Gay WA Jr, Laragh JH: Hemodynamic characteristics of hypertension after coronary bypass surgery and effects of converting enzyme inhibitor. Am J Cardiol 43:586-93, 1979.
33. Malliani A, Brown AM: Reflexes arising from coronary receptors. Brain Res 24:352-5, 1970.
34. Peterson F, Brown AM: Pressor reflexes produced by stimulation of efferent fibers in the cardiac sympathetic nerves of the cat. Circ Res 28:605-10, 1971.
35. Liard JF, Tarazi RC, Manger WM: Hemodynamic and humoral characteristics of hypertension induced by prolonged stellate ganglion stimulation in conscious dogs. Circ Res 36:455-64, 1975.
36. Tarazi RC, Estafanous FG, Fouad FM: Unilateral stellate block in the treatment of hypertension after coronary artery surgery. Implications of a new therapeutic approach. Am J Cardiol 42:1013-3018, 1978.
37. Hoar PF, Hickey RF, Ullyot DG: Systemic hypertension following myocardial revascularization. A method of treatment using epdural anesthesia. J Thorac Cardiovasc Surg 71:859-64, 1976.
38. Brazier J, Cooper N, Buckberg GD: The adequacy of subendocardial oxygen delivery: the interaction of determinants of flow, arterial oxygen content and myocardial oxygen need. Circulation 49:968-77, 1974.

THE COAGULATION SYSTEM: WHAT WE MONITOR AND HOW

D. DAVID GLASS, M. D.

Coagulation Mechanism:

An understanding of the normal mechanism of coagulation and the body's defense mechanisms to prevent excessive coagulation is an essential basis for the understanding of the use of anticoagulants in cardio-pulmonary bypass. There are three main components to normal coagulation: the vasculature, platelets and the coagulation cascade. These all participate in an interrelated fashion in normal hemostasis.

The Vasculature:

An interruption of vascular integrity is the major cause of bleeding in the cardiac surgical patient. The maintenance of vascular integrity is not the only role, however, that the vascular bed plays in hemostasis. Interruption of the endothelium of the vascular bed is one of the important mechanisms for the activation of the other two components of coagulation: platelets and the circulating procoagulants. Exposed sub-endothelial collagen is a potent source of activation of these two remaining components of normal coagulation.

Platelets:

For many years it was believed that adequacy of platelet function in the coagulation scheme was determined by adequate numbers of circulating platelets ($>100,000$ mm^3). Recently, however, emerging concepts of platelet function, not simply the number in circulation, are clearly showing that platelets are a multifaceted, metabolically active component of blood and the coagulation mechanism.[1,2]

Platelets undergo not only an adhesion to damaged endothelial walls, but in addition, release contents contained in vesicles of the platelet which accelerate further platelet aggregation and the development of a platelet plug. The chemical mediator involved in platelet release and subsequent aggregation appears to be adenosine-diphosphate (ADP). When platelets are exposed to storage pool ADP a variety of metabolic functions are activated. The amount of ADP is regulated by two prostaglandins, one originating in the platelet (thromboxane A_2) and one in the vascular endothelium (prostacyclin PGI$_2$). Thromboxane A_2 increases ADP release and is synthesized in the cell membrane of a platelet from its precurser arachidonic acid. This stimulates the platelet to release more ADP and further propagate platelet aggregation and subsequent release.

Inhibition of ADP release in platelets is under the control of prosta- cyclin (PGI$_2$). The substance, synthesized by endothelial calls from the precurser, arachidonic acid, reduces the amount of ADP release and sub- sequently prevents platelet activation. Also, contained within plate- lets and released at the time of activation is platelet Factor III which, along with calcium, appears responsible for the integration and activ- ation of the coagulation cascade. Many platelet activities are under the control of calcium. Both the secretory process and aggregation mechanisms are mediated by the presence of the calcium ion. It may be that the ultimate control mechanism for platelet aggregation and release is under the influence of cyclic AMP concentration. A decrease in cyclic AMP, which can be mediated by increased concentrations of APD, stimulates platelet aggregation. Substances such as prostacyclin (PGI$_2$), which increase cyclic AMP levels, mediate their inhibitory effect on platelets through this mechanism.[3,4]

FIGURE 1:

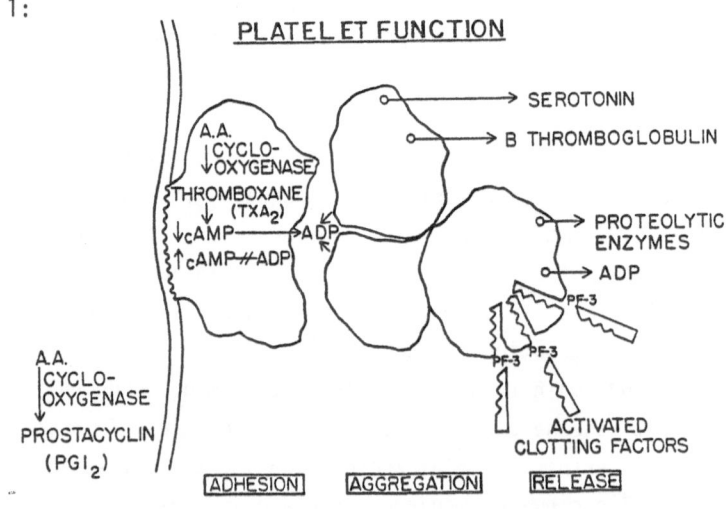

PLATELET FUNCTION

The influence of compounds with vascular as well as hemostatic activity (PGI_2 and TXA_2) on platelet function is important in hemostasis and cardiac surgery. Several studies have recently been done to relate platelet activation and the liberation of these compounds to vascular changes in patients with cardiac disease. Lewy[5] and Sobel[6] have found thromboxane B_2 (the metabolite of thromboxane A_2) in the peripheral blood and coronary sinus blood of patients with vasotonic angina. Robertson[7] also found levels of thromboxane B_2 to be markedly elevated at the time of cardiac ischemia. Preventing this release by antiplatelet drugs, though did not diminish the clinical findings of angina. Propranalol, commonly used as a beta blocking drug in patients with cardiac disease, has also been shown to have inhibitory actions on platelet aggregation and release. This effect is mediated not by beta blockade, but by inter-ference with calcium activation of platelet function and may be part of the beneficial action of patients with ischemic heart disease since it prevents abnormal platelet aggregation and coronary thrombosis or spasm.[8]

Shortened platelet survival in patients with prosthetic heart valves[9] and with coronary graft occlusion following cardiac revasculariz-ation surgery[10] also indicates a relationship between platelet activation in valvular and coronary vascular disease. Other studies are now looking at antiplatelet therapy and have encouraging preliminary results[11] in the prevention of recurrent myocardial infarction.

The Coagulation Cascade:

The third component of normal coagulation is the circulating pro-coagulant factors known collectively as the coagulation cascade. The factors making up the coagulation cascade are in Figure 2. The coagul-ation factors circulate in an inactive form and are activated by one of two main mechanisms. The first is the activation of the intrinsic path-way of coagulation which begins by the activation of Factor XII. It occurs under the influence of a variety of substances: platelet Factor III, antigen antibody complexes and perhaps endotoxin as well. The extrinsic pathway of coagulation is mediated by tissue phospholipid which is released from the cell membranes of injured tissues. Calcium is necessary for both of these route of activation. The final common path-way is the activation of circulating inactive Factor X. Following acti-vation of Factor X, prothrombin is converted to thrombin with a coenzyme, Factor V. Thrombin then cleaves the fibrinogen molecule to form the

fibrin monomer and two fibrinopeptides (fibrinopeptide A and fibrinopeptide B). Polymerization of the monomer and stabilization of the polymerized fibrin by Factor XIII is the final step in the formation of the
tight, firm clot.

FIGURE 2:

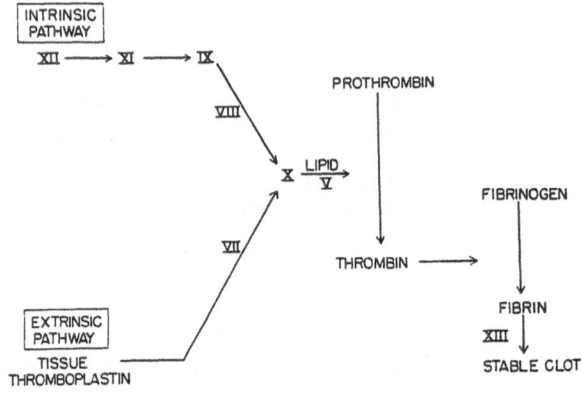

THE CIRCULATING PROCOAGULANTS

The presence of the fibronopeptides A and B not only indicates
activation of the circulating pathway of coagulation, but are physiologically active compounds leading, in experimental animals, to changes in
pulmonary blood flow, heart rate and vascular resistance.[12]

It is important to understand the function and structure of each of
the substances in the coagulation cascade, since they are analogous to a
chain reaction. The coagulation process is one of biologic amplification
which can yield many molecules of the fibrin monomer with a few molecules
of the activated procoagulant precursors. Also, the structure of the
activated procoagulant factors is important in understanding the mechanism of action of anticoagulants such as heparin and the interrelation-
ship of the clotting mechanism to other circulating factors, particularly
those of the immunologic system. The circulating procoagulant factors,
except for Factors I, V, and VIII, are serine proteases and, as such are
protein-cutting enzymes. Each of the factors are unique from one another
by the variability of their inactive form and of the amino acid sequence
of the activated form. However, they all possess a serine moiety which
is the active protein cleaving fraction.

Intrinsic Defense Mechanisms:

As blood circulates in the intact organism, it is essentially inert
with regard to clotting. This lack of activity, of course, is absolutely

necessary or one would otherwise be confronted with the constant development of thrombi. The defense mechanisms for prevention of ongoing coagulation are of critical importance in the cardiac surgical patient. If
they are inhibited in any way then unopposed coagulation will occur with
resultant microcirculatory thrombosis, platelet activation and an
ultimate reduction, via consumption, of the circulating procoagulant
factors.

FIGURE 3:

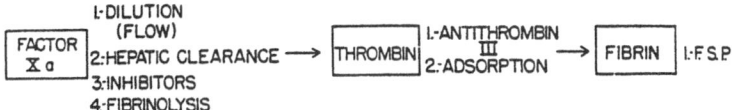

INHIBITORS TO EXCESSIVE
COAGULATION

The primary defense mechanisms present during each of the three
phases of coagulation which are important for the prevention of abnormal
clotting and the preservation of the circulating factors are illustrated
in Figure 3.

The events leading to activated Factor X have defense mechanisms
primarily related to those of flow and the prevention of stasis in the
circulation and hepatic degradation. Adequate cardiac output and reduced
systemic vascular resistance, especially in the microcirculatory bed,
prevent the accumulation of sufficient amounts of activated procoagulant
factors which could induce the deposition of fibrin.[13] In addition,
maintenance of flow through the microcirculatory bed will delivery to the
liver those activated factors that are present for a rapid and efficient
deactivation. Patients with hepatic dysfunction, therefore, may be
unable to remove activated clotting factors efficiently.

In order to prevent ongoing coagulation, activated Factor X must be
efficiently eliminated once it has formed thrombin from prothrombin.
The two mechanisms involved in the inactivation of thrombin are the
presence of the circulating substance antithrombin III (AT III) and the
ability of thrombin to be absorbed onto the fibrin monomer once it has
been polymerized. In the latter case, if no further activated Factor X
is present, thrombin will convert fibrinogen to fibrin, but will be
absorbed on the monomer and promptly yield decreased levels of

circulating thrombin. Antithrombin III is an efficient mechanism to eliminate circulating levels of thrombin when it is present. In addition, antithrombin, because it is a serine protease inhibitor will neutralize activated procoagulant factors that are serine proteases in other places in the coagulation system, as well. It is the only circulating protein whose concentration has been directly correlated with thrombotic diathesis. For the cardiac surgical patient antithrombin III's primary role may be, however, that it is the substance which is necessary to combine with heparin for heparin to be an active anticoagulant (see below).

The final defense mechanism present is the ability of the body to lyse clots once they have occurred. The substance responsible for clot lysis is plasmin. Plasmin is derived from it circulating inactive pre- curser, plasminogen. Plasmin can be activated from plasminogen by an extrinsic or intrinsic route. Activated Factor XII is a potent stimulus to plasmin activation from plasminogen, but tissue activators as well can promote the conversion of plasminogen to plasmin. Plasmin, being only slightly different from thrombin in its chemical composition, and being a serine protease, is capable of breaking apart the fibrin monomer into soluble fibrin-split products (FSP). The products of clot lysis will function as anticoagulants by their propensity to inhibit thrombin and can be used as indicators of clot formation in the same way as fibrino- peptides indicate the presence of abnormal clotting. In addition, they can be used as indicators of clot lysis in both normal and pathologic states. Drugs such as streptokinase and urokinase which are used to dissolve clots in pathologic states function by the activation of plasmin (see Fibronolysis).

Monitoring the Coagulation System:

It is important to have a thorough understanding of available tests and what they determine when evaluating the bleeding patient. Currently, best evidence suggest that when bleeding is in excess of 300 ml/hr, and coagulation tests that evaluate the major components of the coagulation system are normal, re-exploration be undertaken as promptly as possible. The following are examples of coagulation tests designed to define a defect, if present, and the therapy appropriate for that defect. Since no single test will detect all aspects of the coagulation system, several must be performed concomitantly to assess each part of the coagulation cascade. A recent review of coagulation by Fischbach and Fogdall discusses the coagulation system and the tests used to identify defects.

Intrinsic Pathway Tests:
1. Activated clotting time: normal values, 90-130 seconds.
2. Activated partial thromboplastin time: normal values, 25-39 seconds.

The most common abnormality demonstrated by these tests in the cardiac surgical patient is induced by the presence of excess heparin. Infusion of heparin containing blood or the potential reappearance of heparin in the circulation (heparin rebound) will create abnormalities in the above tests. However, a dilutional reduction of circulating factors below 30-40 percent of normal levels will produce abnormalities in these tests as well. The final common pathway is tested, since the end point of both of these tests is the formation of a clot. Therefore, the presence of Coumadin and inadequate fibrinogen may also yield abnormal values.

Extrinsic Pathway Tests:
1. Prothrombin time: normal values, 11-13 seconds.

The prothrombin time, in addition to measurement of the extrinsic pathway for the activation Factor X_A, also evaluates the final common pathway. Therefore, although this is the most frequently done test for Coumadin effect, heparin and factor depletion will also prolong the prothrombin time.

Tests of the Final Common Pathway:
1. Thrombin time: normal values, 9-12 seconds (may be up to 15 seconds in some laboratories).
2. Reptilase time: normal values, 14-21 seconds.
3. Fibronogen (quantitive): normal values, 160-350 mg %.

The thrombin time is probably the most sensitive indicator of the presence of a circulating anticoagulatant. As such, it is prolonged even in the presence of small amounts of heparin.

Other inhibitors of thrombin, most commonly the presence of fibrin degradation products (FDP), will also prolong the thrombin time. A normal thrombin time and a prolonged ATT following protamine administration may indicate excess protamine, since protamine will prolong the

APTT, but leave the thrombin time normal or even shortened (see below).

Reptilase will, like thrombin, cleave fibrinogen. Its major use is in the fact that heparin-antithrombin III complexes will not prolong the value of the reptilase time. It becomes important for differentiating the presence or absence of heparin when the thrombin time is prolonged. Both the thrombin time and reptilase will be prolonged in the presence of fibrin degradation products or low fibrinogen.

Below 100 mg % fibrinogen may be inadequate to produce a clot. It is rapidly depleted in hypercoagulable states (DIC). Less-well appreciated is the marked increase in fibrinogen following surgery and trauma. Values in excess of 700 mg % are common in stress patients. A "consumption" of half of that fibrinogen can occur in hypercoagulable states and still reveal the presence of a "normal" value. Generally speaking, in elevated fibrinogen only occurs after the first post-operative day in cardiac surgery.

Tests of Activation of the Coagulation Cascade:

1. Fibrinopeptides

Normally, none is present. Fibronopeptides are the result of cleavage of fibrinogen by thrombin and indicate the presence of functioning thrombin. Any fibrinopeptide present indicates activation of the coagulation cascade.

Tests of Fibrinolysis:

1. Fibrin degradation preducts (FDP) or fibrin-split products (FSP): normal values: present in a less than 1 to 30 dilution.
2. Tri-F titer, another assay for the presence of fibrinogen degradation products.

Fibrin degradation products are indicative of activation of the plasminogen/plasmin system. This system is activated by tissue activators and the presence of Factor XII. In hypercoagulable states (DIC) clot lysis serves to maintain the integrity of the microcirculation. This is known as secondary fibrinolysis and should not be inhibited until one has dealt with the primary cause of the coagulation activation. Primary fibrinolysis, which occurs without a hypercoagulation, has been associated with post-cardiac surgery bleeding. In this situation, antagonism of the fibrinolytic system may be warranted.

Platelet Count:

Normal > 100,000/cubic mm.

a) Function: template bleeding time: up to 9 minutes in the absence of cardiac surgery; up to 20 minutes following cardio-pulmonary bypass.

b) Aggregation: ADP, collagen and thrombin by platelet aggrego-metry. This is evaluated as to amount of aggregation compared with control.

c) Release: platelet Factor IV:12 to 15 ng/ml; beta thrombo-globulin: up to 25 ng/ml thromboxane B2:0.

Absolute levels of platelets are necessary for adequate platelet plug formation; however, McKenna and Harker have demonstrated that functional platelet abnormalities may be far more common than was once thought. The combination of platelet counts greater than 100,000 and a template bleeding time of over 20 minutes was associated in these series with excessive mediastinal bleeding, which promptly stopped when functioning platelet transfusion occurred.

REFERENCES:

1. Weiss HJ: Platelet physiology and abnormalities of platelet function. NEJM 293(11):531-541, 1975

2. Deykin D: Emerging concepts of platelet function. NEJM 290(3): 144-151, 1974

3. Salzman EW: Cyclic AMP and platelet function. NEJM 286:358-363, 1972

4. Shattil SJ, Bennett JS: Platelets and their membranes in hemo-stasis: Physiology and Pathophysiology. Ann Intern Med 94:108-118, 1980

5. Lewy RI, Weener L, Smith JB, Walinsky P, Silver MJ, Saia J: Comparison of plasma concentrations of thromboxan B2 in Poinzmen-tal's variant angina and classical angina pectors. Clin Card 2:404, 1979

6. Sobel M, Salzman EW, Davies GC, Hardin RI, Sweeney J, Ploetz J, Gurland G: Circulating platelet products in unstable angina pectoris. Circ 63(2):300-306, 1981

7. Robertson RM, Robertson D, Roberts LJ, Maas RL, Fitzgerald GA, Friesinger GC, Oates JA: Thromboxane A2 in vasotonic angina pectoris. NEJM 304(17): 998-1003, 1981

8. Frishman WH, Weksler B, Christodoulou JP, Smithen C, Killip T: Reversal of abnormal platelet aggregability and change in

exercise tolerance in patients with angina pectoris following oral propranolol. Circulation 50:887, 1974

9. Weily HS, Steele PP, Davies H, Pappas G, Genton E: Platelet survival in patients with substitute heart valves. NEJM 290(10): 534-536, 1974

10. Steele P, Battock D, Pappas G, Genton E: Correlation of platelet survival time with occlusion of saphenous vein aorto-coronary bypass grafts. Circulation 53(4):685-690, 1976

11. The Anturane Reinfarction Trial Research Group: Sulfinpyrazone in the prevention of sudden death after myocardial infarction. NEJM 302(5):250-256, 1980

12. Bayley T, Clements JA, Osbahr AJ: Pulmonary and circulatory effects of fibrinopeptides. Circ Res 21:469-484, 1967

13. McInglis TC, Breeze GR, Stuart J, Abrams LD, Roberts KD, Singh SP: Excess intravascular coagulation complicating low cardiac output. J Clin Pathol 28:1-7, 1975

VASODILATORS

MYER H. ROSENTHAL, M.D.

The last ten years has seen an explosive increase in the use of vasodilator pharmacology in anesthesia and critical care. This utilization has principally come in the areas of induced hypotension, control of hypertension and afterload reduction to improve cardiac output and systemic perfusion. In relating this discussion to this course, concentration will be placed on the use of the various vasodilators as afterload reducing agents.

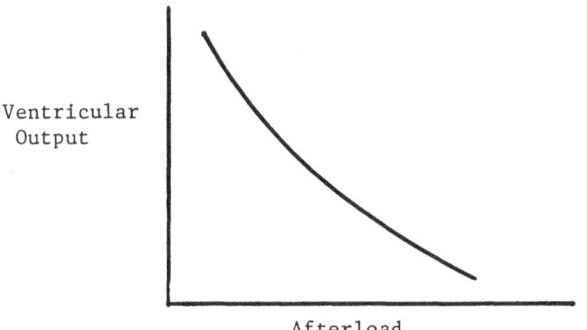

Afterload – the tension in the wall of the ventricle at the time of ejection – is related to ventricular output by the diagram shown above. Since the major determinant of this wall tension is impedance to systolic ejection, in the absence of ventricular outflow obstruction the best correlates to afterload are pulmonary and systemic vascular resistances (PVR and SVR). Thus the calculation of PVR and SVR become the basic monitoring tool for afterload of the right and left heart respectively.

$$PVR = \frac{MPAP - PAW}{C.O.} \times 80$$

Units: $dynes \cdot Sec \cdot Cm^{-5}$

$$SVR = \frac{MAP - CVP}{C.O.} \times 80$$

MAP = Mean Arterial Pressure

MPAP = Mean Pulmonary Artery Pressure

PAW = Pulmonary Artery Wedge Pressure

CVP = Central Venous Pressure

C.O. = Cardiac Output

In administering vasodilator agents the physician must pay special attention to the adequacy of preload as well as the preload response to the vasodilatation. As with endotoxemia or the vasodilator properties of anesthetic agents and adjuvants, the resultant cardiac output to decreased resistance depends on both the ability of the myocardium to increase contractility and the degree of depression in preload. One can graphically examine these responses using either the Starling relationship or ventricular function curves relating afterload to output.

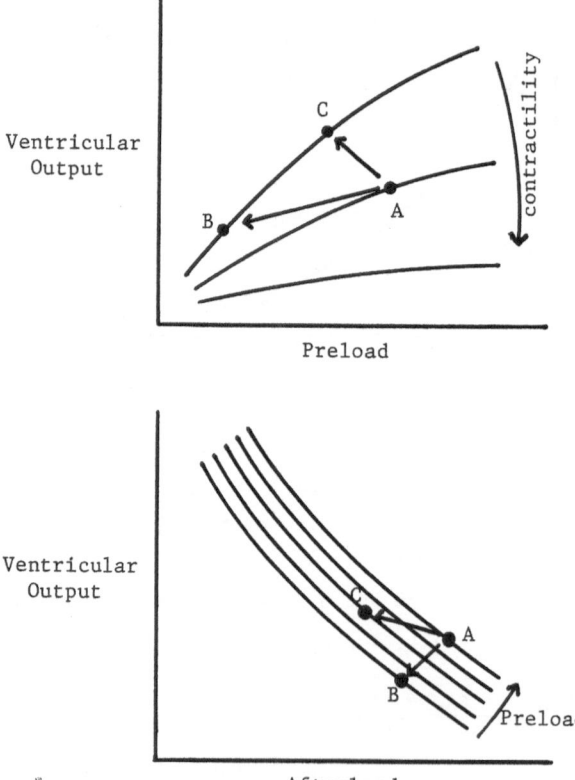

Two responses to a vasodilator given at point A are demonstrated. The result C is accomplished with minimal reduction in preload and thus a favorable increase in output. Point B on the other hand results from a larger reduction in preload; the effect of which is a net reduction in output.

With this as a basic discussion of afterload physiology a few specifics need further elaboration.

SELECTIVE VASODILATATION

The varying pharmacologic properties of the vasodilators allows for some selectivity by the clinician in using the correct agent given the current pathophysiology.

Arterial vs. Venous Dilatation

The properties as regards the arterial and venous dilatation of the commonly used dilator agents vary and this characteristic may be beneficially used depending on the desire to reduce afterload and/or preload.

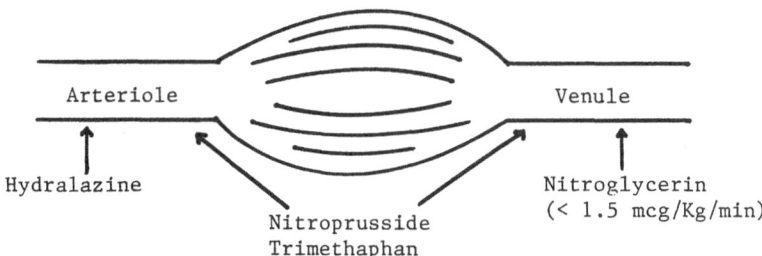

The above diagram demonstrates the areas of selective response to certain agents and non-selectivity of others. Hydralazine with its relatively selective arterial effect is an excellent afterload reducing agent with minimal venous dilatation and thus preload effects. This capability may be particularly of benefit in patients with mitral valve disease. Conversely nitroglycerin in doses less than 1 to 1.5 mcg/Kg/min usually demonstrates predominant venodilatation. This effect may be desirable in patients with hydrostatic pulmonary edema (high preload) who also may have minimally acceptable blood pressure or who may be septic with low SVR. Although generally non-selective in response, nitroprusside is preferred in most acute settings to hydralazine for afterload reduction, due to its rapid onset and brief duration allowing far easier titratability. In certain situations as discussed below, trimethaphan may be preferred over nitro-prusside. As with nitroprusside this agent also is relatively non-selective but shows similar albeit slightly prolonged onset and duration.

Right vs. Left Heart Afterload

Since the recognition of the potential benefit of therapy designed to "reduce afterload", emphasis has, with few vocal exceptions, been directed toward the systemic circulation; i.e., SVR and the left heart. The limit to C.O. has been attributed more to preload as PAW and afterload as SVR since the advent of the flow-directed pulmonary artery catheter. For years Myron Laver emphasized the potential importance of right sided afterload (PVR) with only minimal following. Recent interest in both pulmonary hyper-tension and the hemodynamic sequelae of positive-end-expired pressure (PEEP) has created new emphasis on the importance of PVR and "right-sided afterload" as a major limiting factor to cardiac output. Many vasodilators have been studied, some resulting in short-lived enthusiasm, to provide reduction in PVR. Results have often been disastrous as marked reduction in SVR unac-companied by improved C.O. due to unaffected elevated PVR has led to pro-found irreversible hypotension.

$$MAP = C.O. \times S.V.R.$$
$$\text{If C.O. is PVR limited}$$
$$\Downarrow \quad MAP = C.O. \times \underline{\underline{S.V.R. \Downarrow}}$$

Such results have been observed following administration of hydralazine and diazoxide, two drugs originally felt to have promise in pulmonary hyperten-sion. Additionally deaths have been observed following epidural or spinal anesthesia in patients with pulmonary hypertension. Recent studies have examined the use of nitroglycerin in animals as well as humans with pulmo-nary hypertension of varying etiologies. Most have shown a significant response in reduction of PVR and MPAP following either single dose or infu-sion of nitroglycerin. Previous misplaced enthusiasm warrants some caution in evaluating the role of nitroglycerin for reduction of PVR. However, the safety with which this can be examined in individual patients justifies further use and a cautious endorsement for the consideration of nitrogly-cerin for right-side afterload reduction.

ADVERSE REACTIONS TO VASODILATORS

The pharmacologic properties of any agent include toxicity responses. The vasodilators are no exception yet the enthusiasm for their benefit in reducing myocardial oxygen consumption ($M\dot{V}O_2$) has failed on occasion to recognize potential harm in decreasing myocardial oxygen availability (MO_2 Avail).

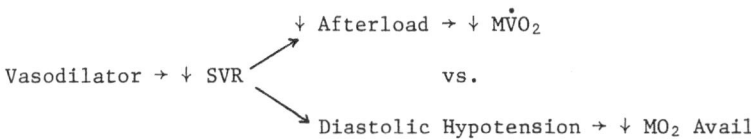

$$\text{Vasodilator} \to \downarrow \text{SVR} \nearrow \downarrow \text{Afterload} \to \downarrow M\dot{V}O_2$$
$$\text{vs.}$$
$$\searrow \text{Diastolic Hypotension} \to \downarrow MO_2 \text{ Avail}$$

The result of the diastolic hypotension in reducing myocardial oxygen availability may produce significant ischemia and arrhythmias. Such sequelae have been observed following administration of both hydralazine and nitroprusside (SNP). Of particular note has been the hyperdynamic response following administration of nitroprusside to patients with left ventricular hypertrophy (LVH)

$$\Uparrow \text{SVR} \; + \; \text{SNP}$$
$$\downarrow \text{LVH}$$
$$\Downarrow \text{SVR} \; + \; \Uparrow \text{C.O.}$$

The response of the hypertrophied ventricle to afterload reduction is often of such magnitude that monitoring for reduction in MAP alone may be both unsuccessful as well as dangerous. Experience has taught that careful attention to diastolic and pulse pressures in the absence of more sophisticated monitors (SVR, C.O.) is necessary to avoid dangerous complications. In the author's own practice, the widened pulse pressure and diastolic hypotension with SNP in patients with LVH has responded either to substitution with trimethaphan for the SNP or the addition of propanolol, both appearing to decrease the hyperdynamic cardiac output response.

Specific pharmacologic toxicity is most apparent with sodium nitroprusside. With high infusion rates (> 3-4 mcg/Kg/min) or total dosage (> 3.5 mg/Kg) concern over cyanide and/or thiocyanate toxicity develops. Blood levels should be closely monitored as well as evidence for decreased oxygen utilization; i.e., metabolic acidosis, and increased mixed venous oxygen content. Thiocyanate toxicity is of particular concern in patients with renal insufficiency.

In summary, the vasodilators have become one of the most useful classes of drugs available to the anesthesiologist dealing with cardiac and other critically ill patients. Work continues to further define and refine their role in managing a variety of pathophysiologic states and in selecting the proper agent to accomplish given ends.

REFERENCES

1. Chatterjee K, Parmley WW: The role of vasodilator therapy in heart failure. Prog CV Dis 19:301-325, 1977.
2. Cohn JN, Franciosa JA: Vasodilator therapy of cardiac failure. NEJM 297:27-31, 254-258, 1977.
3. Fourrier F, Chopin C, Durocher A, et al: Intravenous nitroglycerin in acute respiratory failure of patients with chronic obstructive lung disease, secondary pulmonary hypertension and cor pulmonale. Int Care Med 8:85-88, 1982.
4. Goenen MJ, Leenaert L, Petein M, et al: The effects of tolazoline, nitroprusside, nitroglycerin, isoproterenol and hydralazine on pulmonary circulation early after heart valve replacement. Thorac Cardiovasc Surgeon 30:253-258, 1982.
5. Pearl RG, Rosenthal MH, Ashton JPA: Pulmonary vasodilator effects of nitroglycerin and sodium nitroprusside in canine oleic acid-induced pulmonary hypertension. Anesthesiology 58:514-518, 1983.
6. Pearl RG, Rosenthal MH, Schroeder JS, et al: Acute hemodynamic effects of nitroglycerin in patients with pulmonary hypertension. Ann Int Med 99:9-13, 1983.
7. Rosenthal MH: Physiologic approach to the management of shock. Sem in Anesth 1:285-292, 1982.
8. Rosenthal MH, Pearl RG, Schroeder JS, et al: Nitroglycerin versus nitroprusside in pulmonary hypertension. Anesthesiology 55:A79, 1981.
9. Rosenthal MH, Sladen RN: Mean arterial pressure: a misleading indicator of afterload with sodium nitroprusside therapy. Abstracts Am Soc Anes Ann Meeting, 1978, p. 143-4.
10. Ross J: Afterload mismatch and preload reserve: a conceptual framework for the analysis of ventricular function. Prog CV Dis 18:255-264, 1976.
11. Sladen RN, Rosenthal MH: Specific afterload reduction with parenteral hydralazine following cardiac surgery. J Thor CV Surg 78:195-202, 1979.
12. Stinson EB, Holloway EL, Derby GC, et al: Control of myocardial performance early after open heart operations by vasodilator treatment. J Thor CV Surg 73:523-530, 1977.
13. Tinker JH, Michenfelder JD: Sodium nitroprusside. Anesthesiology 45: 340-354, 1976.
14. Rouby JJ, Gory G, Bourrelli B, et al: Resistance to sodium nitroprusside in hypertensive patients. CCM 10:301-304, 1982.

DRUG THERAPY COMING OFF BYPASS
JOHN H. TINKER, M.D.

INTRODUCTION

Emergence from pulmonary bypass is perhaps the most hazardous period for any patient undergoing cardiac surgery. The success with which the patient can be separated from the bypass machine depends on a complex interaction of factors such as including the success or lack of success with myocardial preservation during aorta crossclamp, the degree to which the cardiac procedure itself has an immediate benefit or lack of it, and the skill with which the cardiovascular/anesthesia team can manipulate hemodynamics during this critical period. In today's cardiac operating room, virtually every case is done with complete occlusion of the aorta, and "myocardial preservation" with "cardioplegia". During the period of aortic crossclamp, myocardial damage may be progressive and severe and will obviously go totally unrecognized. Myocardial damage may occur because of inadequate washing out of the cardioplegic solution (this needs to be done approximately every thirty minutes). It may also occur because of inadequate distribution of the cardioplegic solution secondary to the patient's major disease itself, namely severe coronary artery disease. Extensive myocardial damage may also occur because of inadequate external maintenance of hypothermia and lack of realization that there is extensive heat transfer to the myocardium from the operating room lights and other parts of its environment.

It is very likely that the adequacy of myocardial protection during aorta crossclamp is the single most important factor with respect as to whether or not the patient will be able to be successfully separated from bypass. If this is so, then the problem of predicting which patient will and which patient will not require extensive drug therapy and/or balloon counterpulsator pump management post bypass is a difficult one. Most anesthetists base their anticipation of difficulties on the extent of disease, the patient's preoperative cardiac status especially with respect to the presence or absence of congestive failure, etc. Nonetheless, all too often, we are surprised to find that a patient who should have done well does not and we must scramble for drugs, etc. Some anesthetists obviate this problem by always having available large collections of inotropes and vasodilators already prepared ahead of time. In most cardiac OR's, this is a wasteful practice because of the fact that few patients will require such therapy. Clearly, in a patient with extensive preoperative congestive failure, or a patient in whom there has been extensive difficulties and bypass time is long, or a patient with severe and extensive distal coronary artery disease, preemergence anticipation of difficulties, with anticipatory preparation of inotropes and vasodilators make sense.

MAKING THE DECISION TO USE INOTROPES

Emergence from cardiopulmonary bypass is in essence the replacement of the hydraulic workload on the myocardium. This is done, of course, by clamping the venous return line, hopefully gradually, and, in essence, keeping the arterial inflow pump running, thereby transfusing the patient. If this is being done in your hospital without any form of monitoring, other than the surgeon's "educated finger" on the left atrium or, more usually, the interatrial groove, then I believe that the anesthetist should insist on some more accurate form of monitoring. This can either be a pulmonary catheter, or direct liftage or line or at least a temporary needle attached to a strain gauge with the needle being placed in the left atrium. Coming off bypass measuring right atrium pressure only in a patient whose critical ventricle is the left is entirely unacceptable to this author. Assuming that there is accurate knowledge of either left atrial or pulmonary artery diastolic or wedge pressure, these should be allowed to increase gradually during transfusion to come off bypass.

Most clinicians try not to exceed 15 mmHg on directly measured left atrial pressure, which would be equivalent to a pulmonary diastolic pressure of somewhere in the neighborhood of 22 mmHg in many of these patients. Obviously, if adequate arterial pressure is achieved at less preload than the above, then this should be sought for. Stretching the ventricle by excessive preload input in order to "avoid" inotrope and vasodilator therapy makes little sense because of the fact that subendocardial blood flow is so dreadfully compromised by this maneuver. Some surgeons, even today, insist on rapid massive transfusion up to some arbitrary predetermined left atrial pressure. Very few pumps can readily accept such a massive workload placed so abruptly. This is analogous to dropping a barbell from a ten-foot height onto your shoulders versus permitting the weightlifter to gradually assume the load.

Assuming that the transfusion has been gradual, and that the load that is being placed is reasonable, the decision that needs to be made is whether or not the myocardium is accepting the load. Generation of arterial pressure is an important aspect of this. Many anesthetists go immediately to repeated determinations of cardiac output in order to make this decision. Hydraulic workload is pressure (x) flow and it is pressure which "costs" the myocardium the most in terms of oxygen consumption. Therefore, it makes much more sense to this author to be more concerned about the generation of pressure at a reasonable workload than flow. The measurement of cardiac output at this point in a critically ill patient is essential, however, in order to determine a reasonably adequate peripheral vascular resistance. In other words, someone whose pressure is not above 80 mmHg at a left atrial pressure of 15 or 18 mmHg, may be in severe trouble from a low output situation, but it is also possible that the peripheral vascular resistance is very low, the output is very high, and that the patient will respond to a mere "whiff" of a vasal restrictor. Please note again that I am not advocating the use of vasoconstrictors at this stage without sure knowledge that the problem is normal or even high output with low peripheral vascular resistance. Unfortunately, this is not usually the case. Usually, when the arterial pressure is not above 80 mmHg with a left atrial pressure of 15 to 18 mmHg, the problem is pump failure for one or a combination of the reasons mentioned above.

Although we would not advocate exact numerical limits for such a definition, in practice, patients who cannot generate 80 mmHg arterial pressure or more despite accurately measured (this implies calibration) left atrial pressures of 15 to 18 mmHg, are usually at the "decision point" and will require some form of therapy (see below).

DRUG THERAPY

When the "decision point" mentioned above is reached, it is important to have a logical sequence of treatments in mind. Many anesthetists will start dopamine at this point because it may be better able to preserve renal blood flow (at least at low doses). If 10-15 μg/kg/min are ineffective in raising arterial pressure and cardiac output without much, if any, increase in preload, many anesthetists will switch early to epinephrine. A reasonable starting dosage of epinephrine is 0.05 μg/kg/min. Often, at this point, because of epinephrine's strong venoconstricting effects, left atrial pressure will climb alarmingly if the patient is placed on epinephrine alone. Therefore, at this point, we almost always add a vasodilator, nitroglycerin in our hands, to try to counteract this latter tendency to produce alarmingly elevated preloads in an attempt to maintain reasonable coronary perfusion.

The effect we are looking for is a cardiac index compatible with vital organ life maintenance (which is, at this point in time, somewhere in the neighborhood of 1.8-2.0 L/min/M^2). We are also interested in arterial pressure which will have some chance of providing reasonable perfusion past even the most critical obstructions in various vital organs, especially the heart itself. For us, this means a systolic arterial pressure in excess of 80 mmHg.

Other drugs than the sequence mentioned above have been advocated. The drug dobutamine is said to be more "cardioselective" than dopamine and is said by some authors to be less productive of undesirable levels of tachycardia than dopamine. This is controversial and has been disputed and has not been the experience of the present author. In the unusual instance where the right ventricle is the critical ventricle and where pulmonary vascular resistance is too high, a situation seen almost exclusively in the congenital cardiac operating room, there is evidence that dobutamine hydrochloride may be more helpful than dopamine with respect to preventing additional pulmonary vascular resistance increases. There are also advocates of levarterenol, especially when the hemodynamics indicate a relatively low output situation combined with low peripheral vasoresistance (numbers lower than 700 dynes $\cdot$ sec $\cdot$ cm^{-5}, a relatively uncommon occurrence in our experience. With respect to the choice of vasodilator, there is evidence that nitroglycerin, probably because of its primary venodilating effect, is less likely to dilate relatively normal coronary vasculature, thus producing a "steal" of blood away from the already presumably maximally dilated compromised coronary beds. For these patients, wherein myocardial ischemic damage is very likely, we prefer nitroglycerin.

Thus, when our "backs are to the wall" we find ourselves usually administering epinephrine in doses ranging up to 0.2 µg/kg/min plus nitroglycerin, the maximum dose of which has not been determined, and we find ourselves asking in urgent tones for the assistance of the intraaortic balloon counterpulsator.

THE BALLOON

The intraaortic counterpulsator balloon is the only device whereby myocardial oxygen demand can reliably be separated from myocardial oxygen supply. There is no such thing as a reliable inotrope vasodilator combination which can result in an increased myocardial oxygen supply plus a decreased myocardial oxygen demand, i.e., it is unlikely that in clinical circumstances one can reliably achieve a "pharmacologic balloon". On the other hand, the mechanical balloon mentioned above clearly does separate myocardial oxygen supply from demand and should be called for early in the sequence of events described in this chapter. Many anesthetists seem to feel that it is not in their purview to call for the balloon or that calling for the balloon represents some sort of defeat for their pharmacologic expertise. Actually, if the balloon can reduce requirements for epinephrine, renal blood flow can be better preserved. We believe that in this kind of dire circumstance, which should not happen except in a small percentage of cardiac pulmonary bypass emergencies, the balloon can be lifesaving and should be called for early and insistently. To be sure, there is an instance of complications with the balloon, and equally surely, these complications can be devastating. Nonetheless, the balloon can be lifesaving.

SUMMARY

The period of emergence from cardiopulmonary bypass is probably usually the most hazardous period during any such case. Again, usually, the major cause of major myocardial malfunction at this time is inadequate myocardial preservation during the aorta crossclamp, a difficulty which is less predictable than we would desire. There can be no doubt that crossclamp time, plus degree of preexisting ventricular dysfunction are also contributory factors. Recognition of the problem involves the understanding that flow and pressure must be generated. Arterial pressures less than 80 are, in most people's experience, indicative of major difficulties. Termination of cardiac output at this time will rule out the occasional situation wherein the peripheral vascular resistance is too low and cardiac output in fact is reasonable. Most of the time, when the arterial pressure is less than 80 at measured calibrated left atrial pressures between 50 and 18, cardiac output is low and peripheral vascular resistance is high, indicating pump failure. Drug therapy often is begun with an attempt at preservation of renal blood flow via dopamine, but when severe myocardial dysfunction is present most anesthetists turn to epinephrine, often starting at 0.05 µg/kg/min increasing that dose to a range less than .15 µg/kg/min if necessary. Doses in excess of 0.20 µg/kg/min are usually not helpful and may be devastating in terms of dysrythmias, renalvasoconstriction, etc. The venoconstrictor effect of these doses of epinephrine almost invariably leads us to add a vasodilator, and we prefer the primary venodilator nitroglycerin for this effect. At this juncture, we begin thinking seriously about requesting the intraaortic balloon counterpulsator. This is the only way to separate myocardial oxygen supply from demand.

MECHANISMS AND MANAGEMENT OF CARDIAC ARRHYTHMIAS

RONALD L. KATZ, M.D.

FREQUENCY OF ARRHYTHMIAS

Cardiac arrhythmias in the perioperative period in the non-cardiac surgical patient will be discussed. Although there were case reports concerning cardiac arrhythmias in the operating room in the early 1900s (Levy and Lewis 1911-12), it was not until the past 10-20 years that large series of patients were studied to determine the incidence of arrhythmias. In 1962, Dodd and associates reported a 30% incidence of cardiac arrhythmias in 569 patients. It should be pointed out that in this study an oscilloscope was used and that permanent tracings were not made. Thus, it may be that a significant number of arrhythmias were missed. On the other hand, one can argue that if the duration of arrhythmia was brief and not recognized, then the clinical significance is minimal. The arrhythmias observed were slow, super-ventricular rhythms (atrial rhythms, AV junctional rhythm, wandering pacemaker, sinus arrest with supraventricular escape beats) and occurred in 16% of the patients. Premature ventricular contractions were observed in 12.5% of the patients. The incidence of arrhythmias was higher in patients with heart disease than in those without, being 51% in the former and 20% in the latter. It is of interest that contrary to the clinical impressions of many people, there were no significant differences in the frequency of arrhythmias with ether, nitrous oxide, halothane, cyclopropane, or spinal (tetracaine) anesthesia.

In 1966, Reinikainen and Pontinen determined the frequency of arrhythmias in approximately 1,200 patients. They noted that with halothane, 13% of the patients developed arrhythmias during maintenance. With epidural anesthesia, (prilocaine), the incidence was 18%, whereas with neuroleptanalgesia, the incidence was 16%. In addition to those arrhythmias seen during maintenance, arrhythmias were associated with endotracheal intubation and varied from 25-61%, depending upon the circumstances associated with the intubation.

A year later, in 1967, Kuner et al. reported results in patients in whom a Holter monitor was used to continuously record the electrocardiogram on magnetic tape. The tape was analyzed after the operation in 154 patients. Arrhythmias were noted during the operation in 62% of the patients and in 8% of the patients prior to the induction of anesthesia. The most common arrhythmias in order of frequency were slow, supraventricular rhythms and premature ventricular contractions. There were no differences between the frequency of new arrhythmias in patients with or without preoperative arrhythmias. There were no significant differences between the incidence of arrhythmias in patients with and patients without pre-exisiting heart disease. This finding is in contrast to most other studies of perioperative arrhythmias. It may be that the arrhythmic frequency was so high in this study that significant differences were not observed. As has been observed by others, arrhythmias in this study were as frequent during general anesthesia as during regional anesthesia. Arrhythmias were more frequent in patients undergoing operations which lasted more than 3 hours. Perhaps the greater duration of operation was associated with a complicated type of operation and a patient in poor physical status. However, the authors stated that they could find no correlation between physical status and frequency of arrhythmias. This study is, in general, a puzzling one, since it differs from many of the other studies performed.

Vanick and Davis in 1968 published their study of perioperative arhythmias in more than 5,000 patients. They found that the frequency of arrhythmias was the highest (34%) in patients with known preoperative heart disease, but without preoperative arrhythmias. The next highest (27%) frequency was in patients with known preoperative arrhythmias (these intraoperative arrhythmias being different from the ones the patients had preoperatively) and the lowest incidence of arrhythmias (16.3) occurred in patients with no known preoperative heart disease. The most common arrhythmias were slow, supra-ventricular rhythms and premature ventricular contractions. Arrhythmias were less common in patients under 30 years of age, and 20% of all arrhythmias occurred during the first 5 minutes of the induction of anesthesia. There was no difference between the frequency of arrhythmias during halothane anesthesia (17%) compared with regional anesthesia (19%). The incidence of arrhythmias with cyclopropane was higher (25%); however, these authors pointed out that their experience with cyclopropane was limited, and it may well be that this accounted for the somewhat higher incidence with cyclopropane. Certainly, this figure of 25% is significantly higher than in the author's own studies with cyclopropane. Vanick and Davis also noted differences in frequency of arrhythmias in patients on digitalis. The incidence in these patients was 43%, as compared to 17% in patients not receiving digitalis. This raises the question of whether the digitalis per se is responsible for the arrhythmias, or whether the patient's disease is responsible for the arrhythmias. Although it is not possible to be absolutely certain, it appears likely that both were contributing factors. We have observed a higher incidence of arrhythmias in healthy patients placed on digitalis prophylactically than in a similar group of patients not receiving digitalis. However, the differences between these two groups were not great enough to explain the large differences in frequency found by Vanick and Davis. It is therefore likely that the patient's disease is the most important factor.

In reviewing these studies, certain conclusions may be drawn. The reported incidence of arrhythmias is higher when the ECG is recorded continuously than when it is observed on the oscilloscope. A greater frequency of arrhythmias occurs, (1) in patients who have preexisting arrhythmias or heart disease, (2) in patients receiving digitalis, and (3) when the operation lasts more than three hours. Another important point is the adequacy of respiration. Reinikainen and Pointinen (1966) observed that there were twice as many arrhythmias during spontaneous breathing as with controlled respiration. Although the arterial PCO_2 was not measured, it is tempting to speculate that the CO_2 levels were higher in the spontaneously breathing patients than in those with controlled respiration. Several factors may be involved here: during spontaneous respiration an elevated carbon dioxide may cause arrhythmias, hyperventilation with the associated alkalosis and low PCO_2 may decrease the frequency of arrhythmias, and hyperventilation may initiate reflex responses which inhibit cardiac arrhythmias (Katz and Bigger 1970).

Although it is widely believed that the incidence of arrhythmias with regional anesthesia is less than with general anesthesia, the published studies do not support this view. In addition to the studies mention above, Hughes et al (1966), in dental anesthesia patients found a substantial incidence of arrhythmias in patients who received the local anesthetic lidocaine for dental anesthesia. They also observed that the patient's condition was an important factor. In patients with a normal cardiovascular system, arrhythmias frequency was 17%, while in patients with known heart disease, it was 33%.

ANESTHETIC AGENT

Arrhythmias may be due to the anesthetic agent itself (Katz and Bigger 1970). Indeed, halopropane and teflurane can produce cardiac arrhythmias in concentrations needed for clinical anesthesia (Stephen and North 1964, Katz 1965, Artusio et al 1967). Because of this fact, neither of these agents is available today. There are other agents, such as cyclopropane and trichlorethylene (Lurie et al 1958, Waters et al 1943) which produce arrhythmias, but usually only when given in concentrations greater than needed for surgical anesthesia. With these agents, it is usually possible to decrease the concentration to a point at which the patient is still adequately anesthetized, but without arrhythmias. Of the more commonly used agents such as halothane, enflurane and nitrous oxide, arrhythmias are much less common, even in the presence of an excessive depth of anesthesia. In studies of the mechanisms of arrhythmias with halopropane and cyclopropane, it was clear that there was an important central nervous system component to the arrhythmia (Katz 1966); a finding similar to that of Beattie et al (1928) with chloroform.

ANESTHETIC AGENT AND CARBON DIOXIDE

Perhaps the most common cause of arrhythmias in the past was the combination of the anesthetic agent and carbon dioxide. There have been a number of studies in which the level of arterial PCO_2 needed to produce arrhythmias has been determined. With cyclopropane, the threshold arterial PCO_2 required is 58 torr with a range of 44 to 72 torr (Price et al 1958). In another study by the same group (Lurie et al 1958), the threshold arterial PCO_2 for arrhythmias was 74 torr with a range of 44 to 107 torr. It is known that the threshold PCO2 needed to produce arrhythmias is inversely related to the concentration of cyclopropane.

In studies with halothane, the threshold arterial PCO2 required to produce arrhythmias is 92 torr with a range of 60-140 torr (Black et al. 1959). In a recent study by Eicard and Skovsted (1976), the carbon dioxide arrhythmias threshold for halothane was compared with that of fluroxene. These workers observed a mean threshold with halothane of 97 torr with a range of 82-109 torr. It was not possible with fluroxene to find an arrhythmia threshold. The mean PCO2 achieved in the fluroxene groups was 108 with a a range of 92-115. It is also not possible to demonstrate an arrhythmia threshold PCO2 level for enflurane.

In animal studies of the mechanism of anesthetic agent-carbon dioxide arrhythmias, it was clearly demonstrated that the sympathetic nervous system played a major role in the genesis of arrhythmias. It is well established than an elevated arterial PCO2 can increase plasma cate-cholamine levels. Furthermore, beta adrenergic blockade abolishes these arrhythmias. In addition, treatment such as reserphine, bilateral adrenalectomy or a variety of measures which decrease sympathetic outflow and release of catecholamines prevents the arrhythmias (Katz 1966, Katz and Bigger 1970).

Hypoxia can lead to the release of catecholamines and cardiac arrhythmias. The interaction of anesthetic agent and hypoxia in the production of cardiac arrhythmias has been little studied.

ANESTHETIC AGENT AND CATECHOLAMINES

At one time the most common cause of arrhythmias was a combination of an anesthetic agent and respiratory acidosis. However, the situation has probably changed in the past 10 years. The marked emphasis on maintaining adequate ventilation has markedly diminished the frequency of respiratory acidosis during anesthesia. The wide availablity of arterial blood gases during operations has made it possible to assure that respiratory acidosis does not occur. Although there have been great gains in diminishing the frequency of anesthetic agent-carbon dioxide arrhythmias, the situation is less promising for arrhythmias due to the interaction of an anesthetic agent and catecholamines. This interaction of anesthetic agents and adrenergic drugs to produce cardiac arrhythmias was reviewed 10 years ago (Katz and Epstein 1968). This paper will summarize the information contained in that review as well as discuss some of the newer data available. It is well established that if sufficiently large doses of catecholamines such as epinephrine, norepinephrine and isoproterenol are injected in unanesthetized patients or animals, cardiac arrhythmias will occur. It is also well-known that in the presence of halogenated hydrocarbons or cyclopropane, the dose of catecholamines required to produce an arrhythmia is markedly diminished. The decrease in dose may be as little as one-tenth of the control dose required to produce arrhythmias. This phenomenon is referred to as myocardial sensitization. It is not uncommon to inject catecholamines or adrenergic drugs intravenously for vasopressor effect or bronchodilator effect, or to inject these agents locally to produce vasoconstriction. The anesthetic agents which decrease the arrhythmia dose of catecholamines (produce sensitization) include trichloroethylene, ethyl chloride, cyclopropane, halothane, chloroform, methoxyflurane and fluroxene. These agents are listed in order of decreasing sensitization in dogs. It is known, however, that there are differences between dog and man. For example, trichloroethylene is a more potent sensitizer than cyclopropane in the dog, but in man the reverse is true.

In addition to epinephrine, norepinephrine, isoproterenol, other adrenergic drugs capable of producing arrhythmias in the presence of halogenated hydrocarbons include metaraminol and dopamine. It has been reported that dopamine is less likely to produce cardiac arrhythmias in halothane-anesthetized cats than is epinephrine (Katz et al 1967). However, in the goat, Zahed and associates (1977) found that dopamine had no advantages over epinephrine in reversing halothane-induced myocardial depression in terms of lack of arrhythmias. Our own studies suggest that man behaves more like the cat than the goat, and that dopamine does have advantages over epinephrine as well as isoproterenol in terms of its ability to produce myocardial stimulation without causing arrhythmias. A recently developed adrenergic agent which appears to be fairly specific in terms of increasing myocardial contractility, but with little effect on heart rate or the production of cardiac arrhythmias is dobutamine. Further studies are necessary to indicate whether dobutamine will live up to its early promise of being capable of stimulating the myocardium without producing arrhythmias.

Ethrane is a newer commonly-used anesthetic which appears to be as safe as, if not safer than, halothane in terms of the development of arrhythmias when epinephrine is injected. Vidouse (1975) continuously infused epinephrine during halothane and enflurane anesthesia. The total amount of epinephrine infused to produce arrhythmias was 123 ug with halothane and 174 ug with enflurane. These differences were not statistically significant; however, since there were only 6 patients in each group, it may well be that with larger groups of patients studied there will be a statistically significant difference. Lippman and Reisner (1974) and Konchigeri et al (1974) studied the interaction of enflurane and epinephrine and concluded that epinephrine could safely be used with enflurane.

A greater safety margin with enflurane as compared with halothane was observed in the study of Suzuki et al (1976). They studied 32 children who received epinephrine while undergoing cleft palate surgery. Half of the children received enflurane and half received halothane. Fewer arrhythmias were observed with enflurane than with halothane. Although the number of patients is rather small, other observations would support the concept that the likelihood of arrhythmias following injection of epinephrine is less with enflurane than it is with halothane. Perhaps the best documented study in this regard is that of Johnston et al (1976). They studied the effects of epinephrine injected into the oral and nasal submucosa in patients undergoing transnasal hypophysectomy. Their end-point was the dose of epinephrine which produced three or more premature ventricular contractions. The calculated ED_{50} of epinephrine during halothane was 2.1 ug/kg, for isoflurane 6.7 ug/kg and for enflurane 10.9 ug/kg. When epinephrine was injected with lidocaine rather than with saline in halothane anesthetized patients, the ED_{50} for lidocaine with epinephrine was 3.7 ug/kg as compared to 2.1 ug/kg for epinephrine with saline. If it is assumed that the dose equivalent is one-half the ED_{50} to avoid arrhythmias, then the following amounts of epinephrine could safely be given with various anesthetics: halothane, 1 ug/kg of epinephrine in saline, and isoflurane 3.4 ug/kg of epinephrine in saline was safe. When 0.5% lidocaine was used in place of saline, the maximum safe level could be increased 50%. In our own studies in which lidocaine and epinephrine in various concentrations were intravenously infused during halothane anesthesia, we observed that the protection against arhythmias with 2% lidocaine was greater than with 0.5% lidocaine. Thus, it may be that when 1 or 2% lidocaine with epinephrine is used, even larger amounts of epinephrine can safely be given. The argument may be somewhat academic in that with both halothane and enflurane, the amounts of epinephrine normally necessary to produce adequate vasoconstriction is usually less than the amount which will produce arrhythmias. Thus, one can conclude that the injection of epinephrine during halothane or enflurane is safe as long as reasonable amounts of epinephrine are used. However, there is no doubt that the use of lidocaine rather than saline and the use of enflurane will provide a greater safety margin or will permit the use of larger doses of epinephrine. It is important to point out that in the work of Johnston et al., the epinephrine was injected into the highly vascular oral and nasal submucosa. Thus, the doses these authors concluded to be safe may be smaller than will be safe when injections are made into less vascular areas (i.e., larger doses of epinephrine can safely be injected into less vascular areas). On the other hand, these doses will not be as safe when injected into more vascular areas, or particularly when given intravenously.

Our own studies of the interaction of catecholamines with halothane, enflurane and isoflurane (Conner, Miller, Katz 1976), support the lesser likelihood of producing arrhythmias with enflurane or isoflurane. In a patient undergoing anesthesia for removal of a pheochromocytoma with enflurane, it was noted that during manipulation of the adrenal tumor which produced a systolic arterial blood pressure of 250 torr, there were no cardiac arrhythmias observed. This can be compared with our previous demonstration that the arrhythmia threshold for halothane varies from 175 to 225 torr systolic pressure (Katz and Wolf 1971). In this patient, in whom a systolic pressure of 250 did not produce arrhythmias during enflurane, it was subsequently necessary to turn off the ethrane because of bronchospasm. Upon switching to halothane and with the continued manipulation of the tumor, it was noted that arrhythmias occurred at a systolic arterial pressure of 190 torr, suggesting a lower arrhythmia threshold with halothane than with enflurane. Subsequently, the halothane was discontinued and ethrane was given. Once again, it was possible for the systolic pressure to reach 260 torr without the development of arrhythmias. In a similar kind of situation, the authors are also aware of a patient who underwent pheochromocytoma removal under enflurane anesthesia. In this patient, the systolic arterial pressure reached 350 torr, but cardiac arrhythmias were not observed.

In studies in children it has been reported that epinephrine can safely be used with halothane in the following doses: (1) in infants 3.5 ug/kg, (2) in children up to the age of two years, 2.5 ug/kg, and (3) in children greater than two years, 1.45 ug/kg (Melgrave 1970).

Ideally, the use of epinephrine should be avoided. However, it if must be injected subcutaneously for local hemostasis, arrhythmias can be prevented if certain precautions are taken. An epinephrine concentration of 1:100,000 or 1:200,000 should be used. In most cases, it is possible to achieve adequate hemostasis with the lesser concentration. In the adult, a total dose not greater than 10 ml of 1:100,000 every 10 min., nor more than 30 ml/hr are safe with halothane, trichlorethylene and methoxyflurane. If a 1:200,000 concentration is used, then twice the amount of epinephrine can be used. It is, of course, important to assure that ventilation is adequate so that there is no hypoxia or hypercarbia, since these can facilitate the development of arrhythmias as well as produce arrhythmias on their own.

The value of animal studies in determining the interaction of anesthetic agents and catecholamines can be demonstrated by the following observations. In studies of the dose of epinephrine required to produce arrhythmias during cyclopropane anesthesia, it was observed that in the cat the dose was 0.9 ug/kg (Katz and Bigger 1970). Thus, there is a good correlation between studies carried out in cats, dogs and man. However, human studies are the most important when it is feasible to perform them.

Up to now, we have discussed the subcutaneous injection of catecholamines. However, it is not uncommon in dentistry to make an intraosseous injection of catecholamines. Although, in general, small amounts of local anesthetic and catecholamines are injected in dentistry, the amounts used are sufficient to cause cardiovascular changes. For example, Lilienthal and Reynolds (1975) studied the intraosseous injection of 0.9 ml of 2% lidocaine with 1:80,000 epinephrine. This is a total dose of epinephrine of 11.25 ug. They found that this increased heart rate and blood pressure and produced palpitations and a sensation of a tight chest. These cardiovascular signs and symptoms were not observed when the same amounts of epinephrine and lidocaine were injected subcutaneously.

There have been numerous studies of the mechanism by which adrenergic agents produce cardiac arrhythmias in the presence of halogenated hydrocarbons. Among the more important factors involved are the increase in blood pressure and in the increase in heart rate (Dresel et al. 1960, Vick 1966, Moe et al 1948, Murphy et al 1949, Katz 1965, Zink et al 1975). It has been well established in pharmacologic experiments that if the heart rate increase is prevented or the increase in arterial pressure is prevented that the arrhythmia threshold is increased. Since the injection of a pharmacologic agent raises the question that in addition to the prevention of the heart rate or blood pressure response, there may have been an additional pharmacologic effect on the arrhythmia, the role of blood pressure and heart rate has been studied with changes in these parameters being prevented by mechanical means. A buffer bottle can be used to prevent pressure changes and the heart rate can be controlled by crushing the SA node and pacing the heart. In these kinds of experiments, it has been observed that arrhythmias decreased in frequency or were abolished by the lowering of blood pressure or by decreasing the heart rate.

An interesting study of the catecholamines-anesthetic arrhythmias was carried out by Miletich et al. (1978). They studied epinephrine sensitivity in fasted and non-fasted rats. The arrhythmia threshold in non-fasted rats was 10.9 ug/kg of epinephrine. In rats fasted 12, 24, and 48 hours, the arrhythmias threshold during halothane anesthesia was 5.5, 2.2, and 2.25 ug/kg respectively. The infusion of a 10% fatty acid emulsion increased the epinephrine arrhythmia threshold. They raised the question that fasting might cause a shift from a mixed carbohydrate and lipid to a predominantly lipid metabolic response and thus render the heart more susceptible to arrhythmias. They attempted to support this concept by pointing out that in patients with myocardial infarction, an elevated level of free fatty acid correlates with a higher frequency of arrhythmias. While these results of Miletich et al are preliminary in nature, they raise many interesting questions concerning the implications of patients being fasted overnight.

REFLEX ARRHYTHMIAS

Cardiac arrhythmias are well-known to be reflexly initiated (Katz and Bigger 1970). The afferent limbs of the reflex may be activated by stimulation of the pharynx or trachea, traction on intra-abdominal or intrathoracic structures or manipulation of extraocular muscles and carotid sinus stimulation. The efferent limb of the reflex may be sympathetic and mediated by norepinephrine or epinephrine or it may be parasympathetic and mediated by acetylcholine. Various combinations of sympathetic and parasympathetic stimulation and/or inhibition are possible. It is not possible to state in any given case what the net result may be. However, where the net result is either a relative or absolute increase in sympathetic activity, one may expect tachycardia, hypertension and cardiac arrhythmias as seen during tracheal intubation. On the other hand, when the net response is a relative or absolute increase in parasympathetic activity, bradycardia, hypotension and cardiac arrhythmias may be seen. A typical example of this is the oculo-cardiac reflex.

Depending upon the study quoted, the incidence of arrhythmias during tracheal intubation varies from 0-90% (Katz and Bigger 1970). These differences are probably explainable by variations in conditions of the study, the agents which the patient had been given prior to induction, the definition of arrhythmia and the method of recording and analyzing the arrhythmias. Suffice it to say that arrhythmias can be observed during intratracheal intubation and that these are usually associated with a relative sympathetic predominance. These arrhythmias are usually brief in duration and treatment is not necessary. The oculocardiac reflex or, more properly, the trigeminovagal reflex (defined in terms of the afferent and efferent limbs) is well-recognized. Traction on the extraocular muscles or pressure on the eyeball can provoke this reflex, which consists of bradycardia, hypotension and cardiac arrhythmias. The incidence of this reflex has been reported to range anywhere from 30-87% (Katz and Bigger 1970). Although the injection of atropine to block the efferent limb or retrobulbar block to prevent the afferent limb has been reported to be successful in several studies, we do not believe that these treatments should be routinely used for the following reason: it is possible to elicit the reflex by doing a retrobulbar block. Furthermore, Berliner (1963) felt that the risk of complication in retrobulbar block was greater than the risk of arrhythmias. Intravenous atropine, although effective, can itself produce cardiac arrhythmias. Both Mendelblatt et al (1962) and Pontinen (1966) found that although atropine reduced the incidence of arrhythmias, those arrhythmias which did occur were much more serious. In a study by Schwartz (1971) of almost 200 patients, he concluded that although retrobulbar block and atropine decreased the incidence of oculo-cardiac reflex by approximately 60%, the arrhythmias he observed with atropine were more severe and long-lasting than those in the untreated patients. He suggested, and it has been our practice even since then to not treat the oculocardiac reflex prophylactically. Approximately 15 years of experience with this policy has led us to conclude that this is a worthwhile way of handling the problem. We currently monitor the electrocardiogram and if an arrhythmia appears and persists, the surgeon is asked to stop the manipulation temporarily. The arrhythmia disappears and with gentle handling of the eye it does not reappear.

HYPO AND HYPERKALEMIA

Both hypokalemia and hyperkalemia are capable of producing cardiac arrhythmias. Hypokalemia may occur with (1) renal dialysis; (2) anorexia, nausea, vomiting, diarrhea, intestinal obstruction, fistual with drainage of enteric fluid, nasogastric suction, prolonged parential feeding without adequate potassium supplementation; (3) familial periodic paralysis; (4) elevated levels of aldosterone; and (5) diuretic therapy with thiazide, ethacrynic acid, furosemide, carbonic anhydrase inhibitors, and mercurial diuretics (Katz and Bigger 1970). Not infrequently, patients with these problems are scheduled for operations. It is important to raise the potassium to a satisfactory level before proceeding. Although we prefer to raise the potassium to 3.5 mEq/L, we frequently will proceed when the potassium has been raised to and is stabilized at 3.0 mEq/L. We point out the word <<stablized>>. If one is dealing with a hypokalemic patient and potassium is infused, it is fairly easy to raise the potassium to 3.0 mEq/L or greater transiently. However, it one continues to monitor the patient's potassium, it is not uncommon for the potassium to vary markedly and be quite low several hours after the infusion was given. Therefore, when possible, we prefer to stabilize the potassium at a level of 3.0 or greater over a period of 48 hours.

Hyperkalemia may also produce arrhythmias. This can be seen with (1) adrenal cortical insufficiency, (2) untreated diabetic acidosis, (3) renal disease, (4) sickle cell anemia, (5) multiple transfusions of stored blood, (6) diuretic therapy with aldactone or triamterine, and (7) injection of succinylcholine in patients with burns, massive trauma, spinal cord injury, hemiplegia, or paraplegia (Katz and Bigger 1970).

CYSTOSCOPY ARRHYTHMIAS

Kimbrough et al (1975) observed that cardiac arrhythmias were not uncommon during cystoscopy. In a study of 69 men undergoing 191 cystoscopies, there were 36 patients with heart disease and 33 patients without heart disease. Ectopic beats, ventricular and supraventricular, occurred in 76% of the patients with heart disease and in only 16% of those without heart disease. In patients who received general anesthesia, epidural anesthesia, or local lidocaine, frequency of ventricular ectopics was 8%, 14% and 49%, respectively. There were no differences in supraventricular beats between the three groups. This study, along with others quoted previously, refute the widespread belief (particularly among internists) that local anesthesia is the cure for all operative problems in patients with heart disease.

RBB AND LAD

The combination of right bundle branch block (RBB) and left axis deviation (LAD) occurs in 1% of patients. The question arises whether patients with RBB plus LAD (presumably due to left anterior hemiblock or left anterior fasicle block) require the placement of a prophylactic pacemaker in case they go on to develop complete heart block during operation. DePasquale and Bruno (1976) pointed out that the reason for the frequency of this combination is because the right bundle branch and the anterior fasicle of the left bundle branch are both supplied by the septal branch of the left anterior descending coronary. They also pointed out that RBB and LAD was associated with significant myocardial disease. In 27 patients with this combination who underwent anesthesia, heart block did not develop (Rooney et al 1967). In 83 patients followed by DePasquale and Bruno, complete heart block was seen in only 2 during a cumulative observation period of 262 patient years. Thus, it seems reasonable to conclude that routine placement of a pacemaker in these patients is not necessary.

PSYCHOPHARMACOLOGIC AGENTS

Psychopharmacologic drugs used to treat patients have frequently caused difficulties with arrhythmias. The problem of patients receiving monoamine oxidase (MAO) inhibitors and subsequently eating foods with large amounts of tyramine and the resulting hypertension and cardiac arrhythmias is well-documented. Although MAO inhibitors are being used less frequently than in the past, a substantial number of patients are taking drugs and one should remember that vasopressors which release catecholamines that are normally rapidly destroyed by monoamine oxidase will pose problems. More commonly used than MAO inhibitors are the tricyclic antidepressant agents. These post a threat for two reasons: The tricyclic antidepressant agents block the reuptake of catecholamines and therefore result in an increased circulating level of catechol-amines. Thus, patients on tricyclic antidepressants should receive smaller amounts of catecholamines than normal, since they will over-react to these agents. They should also receive smaller doses of drugs which will release catecholamines in order to avoid severe hyper-tension and cardiac arrhythmias. The second problem of the tricyclic antidepressants which the anesthesiologist may have to deal with their use in suicide attempts. In a study by Serafimovski et al (1975) of 68 patients with tricyclic antidepressant poisoning, 57 (84%) had severe electrocardiographic abnormalities. Another problem in treating these patients stems from the anticholinergic belladonna-like action of the tricyclic antidepressant, which may compound the arrhythmia problem and produce confusion and delirium. Brown (1976) has studied the mechanism of arrhythmia induction with tricyclic antidepressants in the dog and has compared a variety of methods of treating patients and animals with an overdose of tricyclic antide-pressants. He concluded that alkalinization was the most effective method of treating the arrhythmias. Usually, patients and animals with an overdose of tricyclic antidepressants had a lowered pH, in the

7.17 to 7.27 range. The administration of 0.5-2 mEq/L of sodium bicarbonate was found to be the safest and most effective treatment. If supplementary treatment was required, physostigmine was the best additional agent to use, because the physostigmine not only had an antiarrhythmic effect, but also reversed the confusion and delirium produced by the anticholinergic action of the tricyclic antidepressant. This work confirms our own observations on the use of physostigmine in the treatment of tricyclic antidepressant poisoning (Katz and Katz 1972).

Another drug used in psychiatry which may produce problems is lithium, which is commonly used in the treatment of depression. Wilson et al (1976), Targedahl and Gau (1972), and Tseng (1971) demonstrated that lithium is capable of producing t-wave changes, sinus node block, myocarditis, and ventricular arrhythmias. A careful history must be taken in patients presenting for operation to determine whether they are receiving psychotherapeutic agents, which could lead to the development of cardiac arrhythmias.

SUBARACHNOID HEMORRHAGE

Subarachnoid hemmorrhage may cause centrally induced cardiac arrhythmias. The sympathetic nature of this arrhythmia was shown by Grossman (1976) who reported that left stellate ganglion block could abolish cardiac arrhythmias in a patient with subarachnoid hemorrhage. Studies in animals in our own laboratories demonstrated that stimulation of the right stellate ganglion in the dog produced tachycardia, while stimulation of the left stellate ganglion was more likely to produce arrhythmias. This observation fits well with the efficacy of left stellate ganglion block in abolishing centrally induced arrhythmias, presumably due to increased sympathetic outflow following the subarachnoid hemorrhage.

INSECT VENOM ARRHYTHMIAS

An unusual cause of cardiac arrhythmia is illicited by the sting of either the yellow scorpion or the black widow spider (Weitzman et al 1977). The effect of the venom on the autonomic nervous system results in increased sympathetic discharge and an increased level of catecholamines. Weitzman et al (1977) were able to document the increase level of urinary catecholamines; thus, these arrhythmias can be treated with beta adrenergic blockade.

MUSCLE RELAXANT INDUCED ARRHYTHMIAS

It has been known since 1958 (Moncrief) that the use of succinyl-choline in burn patients may be dangerous. Since that time there have been numerous articles reporting cardiac arrhythmia and arrest in burn patients receiving succinylcholine. It was not until 1967 that Tolmie et al demonstrated that hyperkalemia was the mechanism responsible for the cardiac problems. They were able to demonstrate a maximum rise in serum potassium of 8 mEq/L. Since then, many workers, including Mazze and Dunbar (1968), Weintraub et al (1969), Birch et al (1969), and Mazze et al (1969) have reported hyperkalemia not only in burn patients, but in patients with massive trauma who received succinylcholine. An increase in serum potassium in patients with tetanus who receive suc-cinylcholine was also reported by Roth and Wuthrich (1969). Cooperman et al (1970) reported that hyperkalemia following succinylcholine may occur in patients with neurological disorders. They observed such responses in patients with paraplegia following spinal cord trauma, hemiparesis, multiple sclerosis, muscular dystrophy and cerebrovascular accidents. Others have reported succinylcholine-induced hyperkalemia in patients with paraplegia due to spinal cord injury (Stone et al 1970) and in the Guillian-Bare Syndrome (Beach et al 1971) as well as in patients with peripheral nerve injuries (Tobey et al 1972). Recently a hyperkalemic response to succinylcholine in a patient with encepha-lities has been reported (Cowgill et al 1974).

The response of the patient with renal failure to succinylcholine is controversial. One position is that the rise in potassium following succinylcholine in patients with renal failure is dangerous and that a depolarizing relaxant should not be used. However, the vast majority of studies have come to different conclusions. It has been reported by Paton (1956) that the normal response to succinylcholine is an increase in potassium of 0.5 mEq/L. Similar results were reported by Stovener et al (1972) and by Dhanaraj (1975). In studies by Koide and Waud (1972) and Miller et al (1972), the succinylcholine-induced increase in serum potassium was no greater in patients with renal failure than in normal patients. Thus, the vast majority of scientists who have studied the subject feel that the use of succinylcholine is safe in these patients. One point of caution is necessary: It has been reported that in patients with renal failure who have received two doses of succinylcholine, the second dose did produce a rise in potassium of 2.8 mEq/L. However, no untoward effects were noted. A similar greater rise after the second dose of succinylcholine compared with the first dose in patients with renal failure has been described by Powell (1970) and Koide and Waud (1972). Although a second dose or a third dose may produce a greater rise in potassium than normally seen after the first dose, the magnitude of rise is still smaller than that seen in patients with burns. Finally, in a recent paper, Powell and Miller (1975) reported that in 11 patients with renal failure three doses of succinylcholine did not produce increases in potassium greater than 0.6 mEq/L. A reasonable conclusion would be that the evidence at this point suggests that the use of succinylcholine is safe in patients with renal failure.

One important observation is that in patients with burns, there is a period of time during which the patient is at greater risk of development of hyperkalemia than at other times. In general, it was believed that the susceptibility to succinylcholine-induced hyperthermia was from the 20th to the 60th post-burn day. However, the period of risk has been found to extend beyond these times. Furthermore, the period of risk with other disorders is not identical to that observed in burn patients. For example, Mazze et al (1969) found that in patients with massive trauma, the danger period extended from three weeks to the lesion being covered by skin. Cooperman et al (1970) reported that the danger period following spinal cord injury was usually less than 6 months, but could be longer in the presence of progressive neurological disease. Tobey et al (1972), who studied lower motor neuron injuries, found the danger period to be a least 6 months. In view of the marked variation in time period during which a patient may develop hyperkalemia in response to succinylcholine, it would be wise in most situations in which there is any doubt to avoid the use of succinylcholine.

In an elegant group of studies, Gronert and associates (Gronert and Theye 1971), (Gronert, Lambert and Theye 1973) studied potassium flux after succinylcholine injection in normal, immobilized, paraplegic and denervated canine muscles. The greatest potassium flux occurred in the denervated muscles, the next greatest in paraplegic muscles, and the smallest in immobilized muscles. These workers observed that a small dose of non-depolarizing relaxant diminished the hyperkalemic response, but did not block it. It is, therefore, clinically important to remember that the prior injection of a small dose of non-depolarizer will not completely inhibit the succinylcholine-induced hyperkalemia in burn and trauma patients and, therefore, it would seem wiser to avoid succinylcholine.

Bradycardia following injection of succinylcholine was reported shortly after its introduction into clinical practice. Phillips in 1954 reported a decrease in pulse rate to 40 beats per minute. Leigh et al in 1957 reported that the intravenous injection of succinylcholine in infants and children sometimes produces bradycardia. Numerous studies since that time have reported bradycardia, sinus arrest, superventricular and ventricular arrhythmias following repeated intravenous injection of succinylcholine in infants, children and adults anesthetized with nitrous oxide, trichloroethylene, ether, halothane cyclopropane. It is important to remember that the response in children and adults differs. Bradycardia in children is often seen following the first dose of succinylcholine, while in the adult this is rarely observed. In the adult, bradycardia is commonly seen following a second dose of succinylcholine, particularly when the interval between the two doses is five minutes. Under these circumstances, bradycardia occurs in 80% or more of adults. There have been a number of studies of the mechanism of bradycardia following succinylcholine. In general, it appears that the bradycardia and arrhythmias are due to stimulation of both the sympathetic and parasympathetic nervous systems. In any given individual depending upon the age, the anesthetic agent and the circumstances of injection, one may get a predominance of sympathetic or parasympathetic stimulation. Schoenstadt and Whitcher (1963) studied five patients who received repeated injections of succinylcholine. There were no arrhythmias in five patients in whom anesthesia was induced with thiopental and maintained with halothane, but there were arrhythmias in five patients in whom anesthesia was induced and maintained with halothane. Furthermore, three of the patients in the latter group, after injection of thiopental no longer developed arrhythmias with repeated injections of succinylcholine. These workers also found that patients who received hexafluorenine did not develop arrhythmias after succinylcholine. Furthermore, patients given acetylcholine did not develop arrhythmias after a second dose of acetylcholine. However, four out of five patients given succinylcholine after acetylcholine developed bradycardia or asystole. These results suggest that choline, which is produced by the hydrolysis of succinylcholine or acetylcholine sensitizes patients to subsequent doses of succinylcholine, but not acetylcholine. Thus, choline is the sensitizer, but succinylcholine is required to produce the arrhythmia.

In other studies of the site of action of succinylcholine bradycardia, Mathias and Evans Prosser (1968) injected small amounts of succinylcholine directly into the common carotid artery and, therefore, presumably into the pressor receptors of the carotid sinus. In more than one-third of the patients an immediate slowing of the heart was observed. It is, therefore, postulated that succinylcholine was able to stimulate peripheral sensory receptors (such as carotid sinus baroreceptors) and produce reflex bradycardia. It is well-known that acetylcholine, structurally similar to succinylcholine, has a stimulant action on pressor receptors and other sensory receptors.

The bradycardia produced by repeated doses of succinylcholine can be blocked by hexafluorenium and by small doses of non-depolarizing agents. Although it is possible to block the response, one wonders whether it is worth it. In our own studies of repeated doses of succinylcholine, the bradycardia has always been selflimiting and brief in duration. Thus, when the need for a second dose of succinylcholine for endotracheal intubation is necessary, it seems reasonable to carefully watch the EKG and be prepared to inject atropine if necessary. However, in our experience, it has never been necessary to inject atropine, since the bradycardia has always disappeared spontaneously in a brief period of time, always less than one minute.

Cardiac arrhythmias following the injection of gallamine were reported in patients anesthetized with cyclopropane by Walts and Prescott (1965). Tachycardia and hypertension following gallamine have long been known. In general, it appears likely that the major mechanism responsible for the tachycardia, hypertension and arrhythmia is vagal blockade. There is some dispute as to whether these effects may also be due to the release of catecholamines from cardiac adrenergic nerves.

It seems that although it is possible in animals to demonstrate cate-cholamine release by gallamine (Brown and Crout 1970) this does not appear to occur in man (Reitan et al 1973). Recently, pancuronium has been demonstrated to be capable under certain circumstances, of increasing blood pressure and heart rate and possibly producing cardiac arrhythmias. The effect seems to be due to a weak vagal blocking action of pancuronium, an action that is much less than that seen with gallamine (in equipotent neuromuscular blocking doses).

SICK SINUS SYNDROME (SSS)

The sick sinus syndrome consists of sinus bradycardia or arrest with or without associated supraventricular tachycardia. As originally defined by Ferrer (1968) it may include sinus bradycardia, sinus arrest, sinoatrial block, alternating bradyarrhythmias, tachyarrhythmias, and carotid hypersensitivity. The disease is sometimes referred to as the bradytachyarrhythmia syndrome in patients who have alternating brady-cardia and tachycardia. The subject has been reviewed by Scarpa (1976). In general, the mechanism is due to a disordered impulse generation in the sinus node or impaired conduction from the sinus node into the atrium. The anatomy of the sinus node is such that the primary blood supply is almost always a single vessel which arises from the proximal few centimeters of the right coronary artery in 55% of cases, and the proximal few millimeters of the left circumflex artery in 45%. It should be remembered that the same artery supplies most of the atria and that this disease has also been referred to as the sick sinus and ailing atrium. Many cases of the SSS have occurred in patients with coronary artery disease. In the series of 74 patients studied by Moss and Davis (1974), 51 were associated with coronary artery disease, and idiopathic heart disease accounted for 34% of the cases. The remainder had hypertension, rheumatic heart disease, congenital heart disease, and cardiomyopathy. Furthermore, digitalis, quinidine, procaine amide and propranolol can all produce an ECG and clinical picture of the sick sinus syndrome.

Equal numbers of men and women are affected with SSS. Although the peak incidence is in the 7th decade, the SSS can occur in children. The brain, heart and kidney are the organs most affected and which give the signs and symptoms. Moss and Davis (1974) reported that 48%

of their patients with bradytachyarrhythmias had cerebral manifestations including syncopy, near syncopy and dizziness. Review of the literature revealed that 75% of the reported cases had these symptoms, such as the 40 of 56 reported by Rubinstein et al (1972). Because of the changing atrial pattern with bradytachyarrhythmias, embolization is not uncommon, and occurred in 8 of 33 of the patients reported by Rubinstein et al (1972). In the Moss and Davis study (1974), 25 of 74 patients had syncopy. The second most prominent organ producing symptoms of the SSS is the heart. Symptoms include palpitations, angina, and manifestation of congestive heart disease. These may be due to tachycardia as well as failure of the heart to develop tachycardia under an appropriate stimulus. Unexplained episodes of pulmonary edema, ventricular failure or angina may be the result of the arrhythmias of the SSS.

The most frequent single arrhythmia in the SSS is sinus bradycardia, reported in 76% of patients by Moss and Davis (1974). A variety of other supraventricular arrhythmias occur, such as sinus arrest, junctional bradycardia, wandering pacemakers, supraventricular ectopic beats, and intermittent sinus arrest. The occurrence of ventricular arrhythmias in SSS is unusual, occurring in only 10% of the patients of Moss and Davis (1974) and none of the patients of Rubinstein et al (1972). The tachycardia arrhythmias of the bradytachyarrhythmia syndrome are mainly supraventricular.

The diagnosis comes from the history, which includes palpitations, angina and symptoms of congestive failure, as well as syncopy. Physical exam is not helpful, but the ECG is very important. Holter monitoring has been very valuable in these patients. Episodic bradytachyarrhythmias as well as other arrhythmias can be documented. When symptoms and arrhythmias concur with Holter monitoring, the diagnosis is almost assured. It should be remembered when attempting to make a diagnosis that no clearcut cardiac etiology may be seen. This was the case in 25 of 56 patients studied by Rubinstein et al (1972)

A diagnostic provocative test is the Balsalva maneuver. Patients with SSS have a normal blood pressure response to Valsalva, but little or no change in pulse rate. They do not respond to atropine. Ferrer states that if 1-2 mg of IV atropine does not increase sinus bradycardia to a rate exceeding 90 per min, and if after atropine sinus node recovery time remains prolonged after overdrive, the diagnosis is made. The most valuable provocative test in SSS is atrial pacing. Pacing starts at 90 beats per min and increases to 150. At the end of the period, the pacing is terminated and the interval (sinus node recovery time) from the last pacing stimulus to the onset of the next t-wave is measured. An even better concept is that of the corrective sinus node recovery time, which is the difference between the recovery interval following tachypacing and the average resting interval.

Patients with SSS may be divided into those who have major or minor syndromes. Major includes cerebral, coronary or low output problems. Minor includes ankle enema, subjective palpitations and an uncomfortable awareness of a slow, rapid or irregular heartbeat. Patients with minor symptoms may be managed with reassurance. Those with major symptoms require therapy. Pacemaker therapy remains the foundation of the treatment. In general, belladonna drugs to treat bradycardia are ineffective. In the study of Rubinstein et al (1972), belladonna alkaloids did not speed the sinus rate on 14 occasions, and in 4 cases, patients were worse because of the side effects. Induction of tachy-arrhythmia occurred in 2 patients and only 2 patients with brady-cardia responded to the chronic administration of atropine. Similarly, sympathomimetic amines were ineffective in 11 cases, and 5 patients were worse because of the side effects or the induction of tachyar-rhythmia. Pacing was employed in 23 of 56 patients, permanent in 18 and temporary in 5 and was the most successful therapy. A special value of pacemaker implantation is that it permits the addition of digitalis or propranolol without the feat of aggravating the brady-cardia. Thus, in most cases, permanent ventricular pacing remains the therapy of choice. If there are no AV conduction disturbances, atrial pacing may be considered, but more likely ventricular pacemakers will be necessary. In the study of Rubinstein, six of the 56 patients studied died during an average following period of seven years. However, in only one case was the death related to the SSS.

ANTI-ARRHYTHMIC AGENTS

There are a number of drugs commonly used for the control of arrhythmias, including procaine amide, quinidine, propranolol, diphenyl-hydantoïn (dilantin) and lidocaine. Although these drugs can be effective in many patients, drug therapy is rarely necessary. If one reviews the above discussion, it should be obvious that in the vast majority of cases, the arrhythmia can best be treated by eliminating the cause, i.e., lowering the concentration of anesthetic agent, decreasing PCO_2 to normal, avoiding hypoxia, or avoiding the injection of excessive amounts of catecholamines. Therefore, in the vast majority of cases, an anti-arrhythmic agent is not needed. In a few cases, lidocaine, 1-2 mg/kg may be given. The circumstances under which this may be useful is where the cause of the arrhythmia is not immediately obvious and one needs to buy time, i.e., 10-20 minutes to review the anesthetic management, surgical manipulation and make appropriate changes changes. In these circumstances, the injection of lidocaine is reasonable. In rare special circumstances, agents such as diphenyhydantoin or propranolol may be of value. For those interested in these agents, their use has been previously reviewed. (Katz and Bigger, 1970)

SUMMARY

1. Arrhythmias frequently are seen even in the well-managed patient undergoing anesthesia and surgery. However, drug treatment is rarely required.

2. With less than optimal anesthetic managment, cardiac arrhythmias can be a warning that the patient is in physiologic or pharmacologic distress and that rapid remedial action is necessary. Thus, the onset of arrhythmia should initiate an immediate evaluation of anesthetic managment and surgical events.

3. In general, slow supra-ventricular rhythms, such as atrial rhythm, AV junctional rhythm and wandering pacemaker are benign and do not require treatment. However, ventricular arrhythmias should be consider a sign of serious physiological derangement until proven otherwise.

4. The electrocardiographic appearance of an arrhythmia does not necessarily identify the mechanism responsible for the arrhythmia or the circulatory effect of the arrhythmia.

5. Most arrhythmias can be explained in terms of an autonomic nervous system imbalance. Sympathetic predominance may occur by an increase in sympathetic activity or a decrease in parasympathetic activity. Similarly, parsympathetic predominance may be either absolute or relative.

6. Arrhythmias may be due not only to changes occurrng primarily in the heart, but also to primary changes in the central nervous system or in the periphery.

REFERENCES

1. Levy AG, Lewis T. heart irregularities resulting from the inhalation of low percentages of chloroform vapour and their relationship to ventricular fibrilation. Heart 1911-12; 3:99.
2. Levy AG. Sudden death under light chloroform anesthesia. J Physiol 1911;42:3.
3. Dodd RB, Sims WA, Bone DJ. Cardiac arrhythmias observed during aneshtesia. Surgery 1962;51:440.
4. Reinikainen M, Pontinen P. On cardiac arrhythmias during anesthesia and surgery. Acta Med Scand 1966;180: suppl. 457.
5. Kuner J, Enescu V, Utsu F, Boszormenyi E, Bernstein H, Corday E. Cardiac arrhythmias during anesthesia. Dis Chest 1967;52:580.
6. Vanik PE, Davis HS. Cardiac arrhythmias during halothane anesthesia. Anesth Analg 1968;47:299.
7. Katz RL, Bigger JT Jf. Cardiac arrhythmias during anesthesia and operation. Anesthesiology 1970;33:193.
8. Hughes CL, Leach JK, Allen RE, Lambson GO. Cardiac arrhythmias during oral surgery with local anesthesia. J Amer Dent Assoc 1966; 73:1095.
9. Stephen CR, North WC. Halopropane: A clinical evaluation. Anesthesiology 1964;25:600.
10. Katz RL. Antiarrhythmic and neuromuscular effects of QX-527 in man. Acta Anaesth Scand 1965;9:73.
11. Artusio JF, Poznak AV, Weingram J, Sohn YJ. Teflurane, a non-explosive gas for clinical anesthesia. Anesth Analg 1967;46:657.
12. Lurie AA, Jones RE, Linde HW, Price ML, Kripps RD, Price HL. Cyclopropane anesthesia: Cardiac rate and rhythm during steady levels of cyclopropane anesthesia at normal and elevated end-expiratory, carbon dioxide tensions. Anesthesiology 1958;19:457.
13. Waters RM, Orth OS, Gillespie NA. Trichloroethylene anesthesia and cardiac rhythm. Anesthesiology 1943;4:1.
14. Katz RL. Neural factors affecting cardiac arrhythmias induced by halopropane. J Pharmacol Exp Ther 1966;152:88.
15. Beattie J, Brow GR, Long CNH. The hypothalamus and the sympathetic nervous system. Proc Assoc Res Nerv Dis 1928;9:249.
16. Price HL, Lurie AA, Jones RE, Price ML, Linde HW. Cyclopropane anesthesia: Epinephrine and norepinephrine in initiation of ventricular arrhythmias by carbon dioxide inhalation. Anesthesiology 1958;19:619.
17. Black GW, Linde HW, Dripps RD, Price HL. Circulatory changes accompanying respiratory acidosis during halothane (Fluothane) anesthesia in man. Brit J Anaes 1959;31:238.
17a. Eikard B, Skovsted P. Effects of respiratory acidosis on the arrhythmia threshold during fluroxene and halothane anesthesia. Acta Anaesth Scand 1975;19:120.
18. Katz RL, Epstein RA. The interaction of anesthetic agents and adrenergic drugs to produce cardiac arrhythmias. Anesthesiology 1968;29:763.

19. Katz RL, Lord CO, Evans KE. Anesthetic-dopamine cardiac arrhythmias and their prevention by beta adrenergic blockade. J Pharmacol Exp Ther 1967;158:40.
20. Zahed B, Miletich DJ, Ivankovick AD, Albrecht RF, Tayooka ET. Arrhythmic doses of epinephrine and dopamine during halothane, enflurane, methoxyflurane and fluroxene anesthesia in goats. Anes and Analg 1977;56:207.
21. Vidouse JP. Intravenous perfusion of adrenalin during enflurane anesthesia. Acta Anaesth Belgica 1975;2-3:94.
22. Lippmann M, Reisner LS. Epinephrine injection with enflurane anesthesia: Incidence of cardiac arrhythmias. Anesth and Analg 1974;53:886.
23. Konchigeri HN, Shaker MH, Winnie AP. Effect of epinephrine during enflurane anesthesia. Anesth and Analg 1974;53:894.
24. Suzuki A, Yanai K, Taki K. Comparison of epinephrine injection during enflurane and halothane anesthesia. Jap J Anesth 1976; 25:490.
25. Conner JR, Miller JD, Katz RL. Isoflurane anesthesia for pheochromocytoma: A case report. Anes and Analg 1975;54 (4):419.
26. Katz RL, Wolf CE. Pheochromocytoma. In: Highlights of Clinical Anesthesiology. Mark LC, Ngai SG, eds. New York: Haper and Row, 1971:55-65.
27. Milgrave AP. Epinephrine with halothane in children. Canad Anesth Soc J 1970;17:256.
28. Lilienthal B, Reynolds AK. Cardiovascular responses to intraosseous injections containing catecholamines. Oral Surg 1975;40:574.
29. Dresel PE, MacCannell KL, Niekerson M. Cardiac arrhythmias induced by minimal doses of epinephrine in cyclopropane anesthetized dogs. Circ Res 1960;8:948.
30. Vick RL. Effects of altered heart rate on chloroform-epinephrine cardiac arrhythmias. Circ Res 1966;18:316.
31. Moe GK, Malton SD, Rennick BR, Freyburger WA. The role of arterial pressure in the induction of idioventricular rhythms under cyclopropane anesthesia. J Pharmacol Exp Ther 1948;94:319.
32. Murphy Q, Crumpton CW, Meek WJ. The effect of blood pressure rise on the production of cyclopropane-epinephrine induced cardiac arrhythmias. Anesthesiology 1949;10:416.
33. Katz RL. The effect of alpha and beta adrenergic blocking agents on cyclopropane-catecholamine cardiac arrhythmias. Anesthesiology 1965;26:289.
34. Zink J, Sasyniuk BI, Dresel PE. Halothane-epinephrine-induced cardiac arrhythmias and the role of heart rate. Anesthesiology 1975;43:548.
35. Miletick DJ, Abrecht RF, Seals C. Influence of fasting on epinephrine arrhythmias during halothane anesthesia. Anesthesiology 1978. In press.
36. Berler DK. The oculocardiac reflex. Amer J Ophthal 1963;56:954.
37. Mendelblatt FJ, Kirsch RE, Lemberg L. Preventing the oculocardiac reflex. Amer J Ophthal 1962;53:506.
38. Pontinen PJ. The importance of the oculocardiac reflex during ocular surgery. Acta Ophthal 1966, suppl. 86.
39. Schwartz H. Oculocardiac reflex: Is prophylaxis necessary? Highlights of Clinical Anesthesiology. Mark LC, Ngai SH, eds. New York: Harper and Row, 1971:11.

40. Kimbrough HM, Crampton RS, Gillenivaler JY. Cardiac rhythm in men during cystoscopy. J Urol 1975;113:846.
41. DePasquale VP, Bruno MS. Natural history of combined right bundle brand block and left anterior hemiblock. Am J Med 1973;54:297.
42. Rooney SA, Goldiner PL, Musa E. Relationship of right bundle branch block and marked left axes deviation to complete heart block during general anesthesia. Anesthesiology 1976;44:64.
43. Serafimovski N, Thorball N, Asmussan I, Lunding M. Tricyclic antidepressive poisoning with special reference to cardiac complications. Acta Anaesth Scand 1975, suppl. 57:55.
44. Brown TCK. Tricyclic antidepressant overdosage: Experimental studies on the managment of circula tory complications. Clin Toxical 1976;9:255.
45. Katz RL, Katz GJ. Surgical infiltration of pressure drugs and their interaction with volatile anesthetics. Brit J Anaes 1966; 27:756.
46. Wilson JR, Kraus ES, Bailas MM, Rakita L. Reversible sinus-node abnormalities due to lithium carbonate therapy. Med Intel 1976; 294:1223.
47. Tengedhal TN, Gau GT. Myocardial irritability associated with lithium carbonate therapy. N Engl J Med 1972;287:867.
48. Tseng HL. Interstitial myocarditis probably related to lithium carbonate intoxication. Arch Pathol 1971;92:444.
49. Grossman MA. Cardiac arrhythmias in acute central nervous system disease. Arch Int Med 1976;136:203.
50. Weitzman S, Margules G, Lehmann E. Uncommon cardiovascular manifestations and high catecholamine levels due to <<black widow>> bite. Am Heart J 1977;93:89.
51. Moncrief JA. Complications of burns. Ann Surg 1958;147:443.
52. Tolmie JD, Joyce TH, Mitchell GD. Succinylcholine danger in the burned patient. Anesthesiology 1967;28:467.
53. Mazze RI, Dunbar RW. Intralingual succinylcholine administration in children: An alternative to intravenous and intramusclar routes? Anesth Anag Curr Res 1968;47:605.
54. Weintraub HD, Heisterkamp DV, Cooperman LH. Changes in plasma potassium concentration after depolarizing blockers in anesthetized man. Br J Anaesth 1969;41:1048.
55. Birch AA Jr., Mitchell GD, Playford GA. Changes in serum potassium response to succinylcholine following trauma. JAMA 1969;210:490.
56. Mazze RI, Escrue HM, Houston JR. Hyperkalemia and cardiovascular collapse following administration of succinylcholine to the traumatized patient. Anesthesiology 1969;31:540.
57. Roth F, Wuthrich H. The clinical importance of hyperkalemia following suxamethonium administration. Br J Anaesth 1969;41:311.
58. Cooperman LH, Strobel GE Jr, Kennell EM. Massive hyperkalemia after administration of succinylcholine. Anesthesiology 1970;32: 161.
59. Stone WA, Beach TP, Hamelberg W. Succinylcholine-danger in the spinal-cord-injured patient. Anesthesiology 1970;32:168.
60. Beach TP, Stone WA, Hamelberg W. Circulatory collapse following succinylcholine: Report of a patient with diffuse lower motor neuron disease. Anesth Analg Curr Res 1971;50:431.
61. Tobey RE, Jacabsen PM, Kahle CT et al. The serum potassium response to muscle relaxants in neural injury. Anesthesiology 1972;37:332.

62. Cowgill DB, Mostello LA, Shapiro HM. Encephalitis and a hyper-kalemic response to succinylcholine. Anesthesiology 1974;40:409.
63. Paton WDH. Mode of action of neuromuscular blocking agents. Brit J Anaesth 1956;28:490.
64. Stover J, Endressen R, Bjelke E. Suxamethonium hyperkalemia with different induction agents. Acta Anaesth Scand 1972;16:46.
65. Dhanaraj VJ, Narayanamurthy J, Sitadevi C, Mohan Rao K. A study of the changes in serum potassium concentration with suxamethonium using different anesthetic agents. Br J Anaesth 1975;47:516.
66. Koide M, Waud BE. Serum potassium concentrations after succinyl-choline in patients with renal failure. Anesthesiology 1972; 36:142.
67. Miller RD, Way WL, Hamilton WK, Layzer RB. Succinylcholine-induced hyperkalemia in patients with renal failure. Anesthesiology 1972; 36:138.
68. Powell JN. Suxamethonium-induced hyperkalemia in a uraemic pat-ient. Br J Anaesth 1970;42:806.
69. Powell DR, Miller R. The effect of repeated doses of succinyl-choline on serum potassium in patients with renal failure. Anesth Analg Curr Res 1975;54:746.
70. Gronert GA, Theye RA. Serum potassium changes after succinyl-choline in swine with thermal trauma or sciatic ner section. Can Anesth Soc J 1971;18:558.
71. Gronert GA, Lambert EH, Theye RA. The response of denervated skeletal muscle to succinylcholine. Anesthesiology 1973;39:13.
72. Phillips HS. Physiologic changes noted with the use of succinyl-choline chloride as a muscle relaxant during endotracheal intub-ation. Anesth Analg 1954;33:165.
73. Leigh MD. McCoy DD, Belton MK, Lewis GB. Bradycardia following intravenous administration of succinylcholine chloride to infants and children. Anesthesiology 1957;18:698.
74. Schoenstadt DA, Whitcher CE. Observations on the mechanism of succinylcholine-induced cardiac arrhythmias. Anesthesiology 1963; 24:358.
75. Mathias JA, Evans-Prosser C. An investigation into the site of action of suxamethonium on cardiac rhythm. Proceedings of Fourth World Congress of Anesthesiologists, 1968, London, 1153.
76. Walts LF, Prescott FS. The effects of gallamine on cardiac rhythm during general anesthesia. Anesth Analg 1965;44:265.
77. Brown ER, Crout JR. The sympathomimetic effect of gallamine on the heart. Anesthesiology 1968;29:179.
78. Reitan JA, Fraser AI, Eisele JH. Lack of cardiac inotropic effects of gallamine in anesthetized man. Anesth Analg Curr Res 1973; 52:974.
79. Ferrer MI. The sick sinus syndrome in atrial disease. JAMA 1968; 206:645.
80. Scarpa WJ. The sick sinus syndrome. Am Heart J 1976;92:648.
81. Moss AJ, Davis RJ. Brady-tachy syndrome. Prog Cardiovasc Dis 1974;16:439.
82. Rubenstein J, Schulman C, Yurchak, Pavd De Sanctis R. Clinical spectrum of the sick sinus syndrome. Circulation 1972;46:5.

ANESTHETIC CARE OF THE PATIENT IN SHOCK

D.E. LONGNECKER

Shock may be classified according to its cause as hemorrhagic, septic, cardiac, or neurogenic in origin. This discussion will consider the pathophysiology and treatment of hemorrhagic shock only. Emphasis will be placed on clinical application of concepts which are relevant either to the diagnosis or the treatment of hemorrhage, but the salient pathophysiological features of hemorrhage will be reviewed in order to provide a rational basis for treatment.

PATHOPHYSIOLOGY OF HEMORRHAGIC SHOCK

Tissue Perfusion

The fundamental defect in hemorrhagic shock is tissue ischemia. As circulating blood volume is reduced and arterial pressure declines, various peripheral circulatory mechanisms are activated which attempt to restore tissue perfusion and prevent cellular hypoxia. One of the important compensatory mechanisms is a redistribution of cardiac output which attempts to preseve tissue perfusion to vital organs. This redistribution results from marked increases in vascular resistance in the renal, skeletal muscle and cutaneous circulations, while splanchnic vascular resistance is moderately increased and cerebral and coronary vascular resistances are altered only slightly. The net result is a reduction in blood flow to all organs because of the reduced cardiac output, but the fraction of blood delivered to the brain and heart is increased at the expense of other organs. The initial benefits of this flow redistribution include the maintenance of cerebral and coronary perfusion, but the consequences are organ failure in other essential organs such as the kidney. The combination of increased vascular resistance, reduced cardiac output and reduced perfusion pressure severely restricts renal blood flow and the result is oliguric renal failure. The splanchnic viscera are also vulnerable to ischemia during hemorrhagic shock and, in animals, the prevention of splanchnic ischemia markedly improves survival following hemorrhage. Even those organs which are relatively protected eventually deteriorate unless the condition is corrected rapidly. Cerebral ischemia is manifested clinically by the confusion and stupor which accompany severe hemorrhage and maintenance of cerebral blood flow results in markedly prolonged survival times in hemorrhaged dogs, suggesting that cerebral ischemia ultimately contributes to the mortality of hemorrhage.

Autonomic Nervous System

During hemorrhage, there is a prompt increase in sympathetic activity resulting in arteriolar constriction in those organs (muscle, skin, and kidney) which are most responsive to adrenergic influences. Circulating catecholamines increase markedly during hemorrhage and eventually contribute to the ischemia accompanying prolonged hypovolemia. The infusion of norepinephrine into hemorrhaged dogs results in increased mortality, presumably by enhancing tissue ischemia by vasoconstriction. Plasma renin activity is increased markedly during hemorrhage also. Pharmacological blockade of either the adrenergic nervous system or the renin-angiotensin system prevents the increases in vascular resistance which accompany hemorrhage and improves the survival rates of hemorrhaged animals.

Metabolic Alterations

There is a progressive decrease in aerobic metabolism and a consequent increase in anaerobic metabolism during hemorrhage. There are at least two major consequences of the shift to anaerobic metabolism: (a) cellular energy production is markedly impaired, and (b) metabolic acidosis results. Normally, the aerobic metabolism of glucose is the principal source of ATP, the major fuel for cellular activity. When cells become hypoxic, pyruvate is converted to lactic acid and ATP production is markedly reduced (to about five percent of normal). As lactate accumulates in the cells it spills over into the blood, resulting in the metabolic acidosis commonly seen during prolonged hemorrhage.

DIAGNOSIS AND TREATMENT OF HEMORRHAGIC SHOCK

Monitors

Essential monitors include measures of central venous pressure, arterial pressure, heart rate, urine output, and blood gases. A monitor of organ perfusion is especially important during hypovolemia, but direct measures of tissue blood flow remain experimental at this time. However, urine output is an indicator of renal perfusion and this is especially helpful because renal vasoconstriction occurs promptly with blood loss. Arterial cannulation provides a reliable measure of arterial pressure and a convenient source of arterial blood. Arterial blood gases and pH should be monitored during hypovolemia, but these values commonly do not reflect the major change which occur in the tissues. Typically, arterial PO_2 and pH remain near normal and PCO_2 is decreased during hemorrhage. In contrast, the tissues are hypoxic and hypercarbic during hemorrhagic shock and these alterations are not evident in the arterial blood. Central venous blood gases do reflect the extent of the tissue hypoxia and hypercarbia accompanying hemorrhage and these values should be monitored during hypovolemia.

Therapeutic Goals

The major pathophysiologic alteration in hemorrhagic shock is tissue ischemia. Ischemia results both from a reduction in cardiac output and from increased peripheral vascular resistance, and therapy should be directed towards correcting both of these problems. Restoration of circulating blood volume is the cornerstone of therapy, and prevention of intense peripheral vasoconstriction is an important adjunct in order to minimize the extent of tissue ischemia.

Fluids

The foundation of fluid volume therapy for hemorrhagic shock is the red blood cell. The amount of blood to be replaced cannot be determined on an arbitrary basis. Rather, the adequacy of volume replacement must be assessed by clinical signs and the monitors described previously.

Balanced salt solutions are also required to replace the total volume deficit, since major interstitial fluid shifts accompany hemorrhage.

Acid-Base Therapy

Persistent metabolic acidosis is almost always an indication of inadequate volume replacement rather than a consequence of blood transfusion itself. Massive transfusion usually results in alkalosis as a consequence of citrate metabolism; not in acidosis, which is an indicator of inadequate tissue perfusion. Bicarbonate therapy should be based on actual blood gas determinations and not on an empiric formula, since the combination of citrate metabolism plus bicarbonate administration results in marked metabolic alkalosis after resuscitation. It is especially important to calculate the base deficit because respiratory alkalosis may obscure the metabolic acidosis of hemorrhage.

Drug Therapy

Intense peripheral vasoconstrictors should be avoided in the treatment of hemorrhagic shock. Steroid therapy has been controversial in hemorrhagic shock, but recent studies suggest that steroids have a role in the treatment of hypovolemia. Steroids prevent the intense arteriolar constriction associated with hemorrhage without producing vasodilation, and the survival rates of hemorrhaged animals are considerably improved when steroids are administered during hemorrhage.

Anesthetic Management

Although there is little objective evidence in humans to support one anesthetic technique over another, there are laboratory data which suggest that some anesthetics are better tolerated than others during hemorrhage. During graded hemorrhage, animals anesthetized with cyclopropane survived for markedly shorter intervals than did those receiving halothane. In rats which were hemorrhaged during anesthesia with one of four anesthetics, the mortality was least in those anesthetized with ketamine. Small bowel and hepatic necrosis was less evident in hemorrhaged rats receiving ketamine, suggesting that ketamine may be of value in preventing tissue ischemia in hemorrhaged animals. Direct measurements of tissue oxygen tension also support this conclusion.

REFERENCES

1. Zweifach BW, Fronek A: The interplay of central and peripheral factors in irreversible hemorrhagic shock. Prog Cardiovascular Disease 18(2):147-180, 1975
2. Longnecker DE, Sturgill BC: Influence of anesthetic agent on survival following hemorrhage. Anesthesiology 45:516-521, 1976
3. Longnecker DE, Ross DC, Silver IA: Anesthetic influence on arteriolar diameters and tissue oxygen tension in hemorrhaged rats. Anesthesiology 57:177-182, 1982

CURRENT CONCEPTS OF MASSIVE TRANSFUSION THERAPY

D. David Glass, M.D.

The exchange of blood from man to man has been recognized for years.
the Old Testament has several quotes upon which the refusal of blood
transfusion is based. Likewise, ancient references to the therapeutic
use of blood also can be found. The Egyptians and Norwegians drank
blood as a cure for such diverse diseases as epilepsy and elephantiasis.
An ancient Hebrew manuscript actually cites the placement of blood from
one man's veins into another.

In 1937 the first blood bank was established, a relatively recent event,
and it was not until the 1960's that the processing and use of components became routine.

Today, the use of components has varied widely because of available,
individual preference, education and regional transfusion practice.

This lecture will focus on current transfusion practices involving red
blood cells, components for hemostasis and blood and blood related
products of potential use in the future.

I. Red Blood Cell Transfusions
    A. Compatibility. Tests for donor and recipient compatibility
        have been recently described in a previous course (Brzica,
        ASA Ref. #125, 1982) and is available in depth (Petz LD,
        Swisher SN, Clinical Practice of Transfusion Therapy) and
        as such will not be reviewed.

        1. Red cell availability for surgical schedules.
            a. Type and screen (hold). This technique is being
                used with increasing frequency for elective surgery
                not usually requiring blood, but which on some
                occasion may be needed. The major advantages in-

clude: 1) reduce actual number of units set aside each day for surgery, 2) less work for blood bank personnel, 3) lower patient cost. A major antibody screen of the recipient also allows for time to identify and have nonantigenic blood available.

b. Maximum surgical blood order scheduling. Develops profile for each individual procedure/institution and reduces excessive crossmatching.

2. Urgent transfusion requirements when complete compatibility evaluation cannot be done.

a. O negative (universal donor) blood. O blood lacks both the A and B antigens and theoretically can be used when typing and crossmatching are not possible. Some dangerous reactions can and do occur.

b. Type specific blood. ABO-Rh type specific, but non-crossmatched blood. Preferable to O and if no previous sensitization has occurred, will nearly always be successful. Two-thirds of Rh negative people will be immunized by Rh positive blood if only ABO typing done.

c. Type specific partially crossmatched blood. Designed to eliminate the potential of serious errors in ABO typing. Preferable to either of the above.

B. Citrate Anticoagulant

1. For many years ACD (acid citrate dextrose) was the main anticoagulant. The arbitrary standard of "70% of transfused RBC's must be recovered 24-hours after infusion" was reached at 21 days in $1-6^{o}$ storage with ACD.

2. Today most blood is drawn in CPD-adenine preservative. Adenine has been added to provide a precursor for ATP synthesis. Maintenance of ATP levels are thought to be the most important factor in lessening RBC deformity. Less deformity means less sequestration and a longer

circulating cellular life span.

3. RBC viability. Preservation of RBC function should also be a goal of storage. The ability of RBC's to unload O_2 at the tissues is regulated by the levels of 2-3 DPG (2-3 diphosphoglyerate). Red cells depleted of 2-3 DPG, release O_2 at the tissue less readily. In ACD blood, 2-3 DPG levels fall to one-half of the normal level after five days; to 25% after 10 days and to less than 10% at the end of the three week storage period. In contrast, 2-3 DPG in CPD-A1 falls more readily than in CPD alone, but is still above that found in ACD.

The importance of 2-3 DPG has been controversial. Recently, however, Weisel has documented low cardiac indices following abdominal aortic aneurysm surgery with low 2-3 DPG (low P_{50}) and an inability of these patients to respond to volume loading in the first 24 hours following surgery. Dennis et al has shown improved ventricular function when 2-3 DPG enriched cells were administered to patients following cardiac surgery when compared with groups receiving routine stored blood. It would appear that 2-3 DPG concentration is no longer a laboratory curiousity.

C. Whole Blood. While nearly all recipients of whole blood could receive pack cells, the pendulum has swung away from the belief by many that only components should be used, to the use of whole blood in some circumstances. Often the cost of whole blood is less than the use of various components and no one can argue the convenience. Storage in CPD-A1 has improved the whole blood product even with prolonged storage.

D. Packed Cells. The advantages to sedimented red cells, which have an average hematocrit of 70% or centrifuged red cells which have an average hematocrit of 85%, are several. Mild blood loss can be replaced with components of packed cells and either crystalloid or colloid for volume supplement. With packed cells, one gains almost double the hemoglobin

per unit volumes as in whole blood. The threat of circulatory overload with whole blood transfusions, particularly
in pediatrics, abounds in the literature. In carefully
monitored patients this should not occur. But certainly,
it is a consideration particularly in patients where only
increasing red cell mass is the therapeutic goal.

E. Washed Red Blood Cells. A saline was of RBC's is done to
remove all of the plasma and most nonerythrocyte debris.
The amount of retained non-RBC's and lost RBC's varies
widely with the technique. The main indication is for
patients with strong allergic transfusion reactions.
Anaphylactic reactions have been reported to occur in IgA
deficit blood recipients and in these patients washed cells
could be used.

F. Frozen Red Blood Cells. Grove-Rasmussen has stated that O
group red blood cells processed in the washed freezing
fashion can be regarded as safe recipient for all ABO
groups. The risk of hepatitis is less, although probably
not absent. Frozen cells were also thought to improve
transplant viability by reducing white blood cell infusion.
However, recent information would indicate that nonfrozen
blood (whole or packed cells) actually improves transplant
survival. Because of the cost of frozen blood and prolonged
shelf life of CPD stored blood, the use of frozen RBC's has
declined in many centers in recent years.

G. Leukocyte-Poor RBC's. White blood cell antibodies are responsible for a significant number of febrile, non-hemolytic
transfusion reactions. This is particularly true in patients that have had large numbers of transfusions in the
past. The presence of leukocyte antibodies may exist in
one-third to one-half the population. Units which are prepared as leukocyte-poor units eliminate between 70-95% of
of all WBC's and have led to an 80% decrease in febrile
transfusion reaction in some centers.

II. Components for Hemostasis

A. Platelets. The level of platelet count necessary for adequate hemostasis has been widely debated. Certainly, 100,000 per cubic millimeter of normally functioning platelets is adequate for surgical hemostasis. Below 30,000-50,000 of normally functioning platelets, there is probably an increased incidence of surgical bleedings. There are two aspects of the adequacy of platelet function. Even with over 100,000 platelets, when antiplatelet drugs, like aspirin, have been utilized there may be ineffective hemostasis. Secondly, it is quite apparent in recent studies that the rapidity of all of the platelet count may also be significant. A slow descent to even 5,000 in thrombocytopenic patients is often well tolerated; whereas, precipitous falls from 150,000 to 50,000 may be associated with bleeding. Platelet storage has also been controversial. It has been recently noted that storage at room temperature for 72 hours is attended by good platelet recovery and life span; however, there is a loss of effective aggregation at the time of administration. In contrast, platelets stored between 1 and 6° C have better acute function, but cannot be recovered in the circulation after 24 hours. Acute bleeding would, in theory best be treated with the transfusion of cold storage platelets, while prophylactic transfusion in thrombocytopenia best with room temperature storage. (Figure 1)

It is now recognized that many coagulopathies in the perioperative period can be shown to be caused by platelet dysfunction. It will be important in the future to establish the best method for procurement and storage of platelets for treatment of perioperative bleeding.

The number of platelets to administer is about one donor equivalent unit of platelets for each 10 Kg body weight to increase the platelet count 50,000/min.[3]

Platelets (and WBC's) can be obtained from single donors by the technique of cytapheresis which eliminates pooled donor packs.

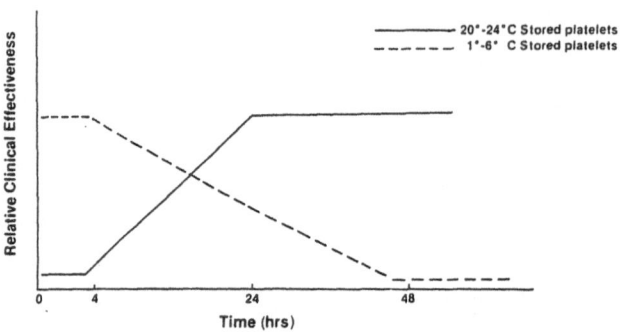

FIGURE 1

B. Coagulation Factors. With the exception of labile Factors
    V and VIII, all plasma coagulation factors are stable in
    banked blood. When it is necessary to replace these fac-
    tors, either for surgical hemostasis or for therapy of
    primary congenitial defects, fresh frozen plasma yields the
    equivalent clotting factors of a single unit of fresh blood.
    There are at present also factor concentrates of II, VII,
    IX, X (Konyne$^{(R)}$ or Proplex$^{(R)}$, cryoprecipitate (I and VIII)
    and specific factors for hemophilia and fibrinogen deficien-
    cies.

    1. Antithrombin III. Antithrombin III is one of the
        primary defense mechanisms for inhibition of the coagu-
        lation cascade. In addition, it is the cofactor neces-
        sary for heparin to function optimally as an anticoagu-
        lant. Recently, ATIII has been used for therapy of
        thrombotic conditions such as pulmonary embolism, hemo-
        lytic uremic syndrome and DIC. The potential for ATIII
        as a useful component is great and further studies will
        be necessary to delineate its precise value. At the
        present time, the only source of ATIII is fresh frozen
        plasma.

    2. Fibronectin. The reduction of opsonic activity in
        patients following sepsis or trauma may play a role in
        the pathogenesis of respiratory failure. Cryoprecipi-
        tate contains high levels of cold insoluble globulin
        which is identical to fibronectin. Recent data of Saba

and others suggest that in addition to fibrinogen and VIII, cryoprecipitate will restore fibronectin levels.

III. Blood Substitutes

The search for an alternative to whole blood transfusion has been sought for some time. Many volume substitutes to whole blood do exist and will not be reviewed here.

Currently only two possibilities seem to exist as an alternative to red blood cells for oxygen transport.

A. Stroma Free Hemoglobin. The renal and coagulation changes seen with a transfusion reaction and the liberation of free hemoglobins caused by red cell stroma and not the hemoglobin. By removing the stroma, the remaining hemoglobin (mol. wt. 64,000) can carry oxygen and function as an oncotically active substance as well.

   1. Advantages include:

      a. No necessity for blood typing
      b. Prolonged room temperature storage
      c. Ideal rhoelogical properties
      d. Especially beneficial in acute volume resuscitation

      Conjugation of the hemoglobin with pyridoxal phosphate reduces renal clearance and prolongs intravascular duration.

B. Fluorocarbons. The fluorocarbons were first synthesized during the Manhattan Project in World War II. The compounds are used as coolants, and in 1966 Clark and Gallan, recognizing their properties of O_2 and CO_2 content, first used them for liquid breathing. Modell and his co-workers have studied several preparations and found the fluorocarbons capable of sustaining life for brief periods when utilized for liquid respiration. Geyer described the fluorocarbons as an artificial blood substitute and showed that rats survived when blood was completely replaced with a fluorocarbon, hydroxyethyl starch solution. Although not perfect and with most of the usual circulating substances absent, life can be sustained, apparently without residual defect, for short periods of time in animals. Possible application includes:

1. Artificial blood substitute.
   a. Pump prime
   b. Emergency situation, especially when blood cannot be given or not available

2. Organ preservation

3. Cardioplegia solutions

Several humans have now received fluorocarbons in Japan and in 1979 the first human, a Jehovah's Witness, was given a fluorocarbon infusion in the United States. The emulsion contained perfluorodecalin and perfluoropylamine. The emulsions can be obtained for certain circumstances such as Jehovah's Witnesses.

IV. Disease Transmission and Transfusion Therapy

A. Hepatitis. The risk of hepatitis transmission continues to be of clinical importance. Testing for HBV (Hepatitis B Virus). Screening for nonA, nonB will also reduce the risk of disease transmission.

   1. Relative Risk:
      High Risk: Pooled plasma derivatives

      a. Factor VIII (AHG concentrates)
      b. Factor IX (prothrombin concentrates)

      Moderate Risk: Whole blood and single unit components of blood or single donor pheresis

      a. RBC - platelet - FFP
      b. Cryoprecipitate
      c. Frozen and washed RBC's

      Safe: Heat treated plasma proteins

B. Other Diseases

   1. Recently, attention has been focused on the transmission of Autoimmune Deficiency Syndrome (AIDS) in several hemophiliacs. This raises the question of acceptable donors in diverse socioeconomic groups.

2. Other disease which may be of concern include:

    a. Malaria, syphilis, CMG virus and Epstien-Barr virus

    b. Other parasites and bacteria

Selected References:

1. Weisel RD, Dennis RC, Manny J, et al: Adverse effects of transfusion therapy during abdominal aortic aneurysectomy. Surgery 83:682-690, 1978.
2. Dennis RC, Hechtman HB, Berger RL, et al: Transfusion of 2-3DPG enriched red blood cells to improve cardiac function. Ann Thor Surg 26-17-26, 1978.
3. Lanser ME, Saba TM, Scovill WA: Opsonic glycoprotein (plasma fibronectin) levels after burn injury. Ann Surg, Vol 192, No 6, pp 776-782, 1980.
4. Scovill WA, Saba TM, Blumenstock FA, et al: Opsonic surface binding glycoprotein therapy during sepsis. Ann Surg, Vol 188, No 4, pp 521-529, 1978.
5. Greenburg AG, Hayash R, Seifert I, et al: Intravascular persistence and oxygen delivery of pyridoxalated, stroma-free hemoglobin during gradations of hypotension. Surgery 86:13-16, 1979.
6. Freola M, Azar D, Wiener L: Improved oxygenation of ischemis myocardium by hemodilution with stroma-free hemoglobin solution. Chest 75:369-375, 1979.
7. Modell JH, et al: Oxygenation by ventilation with fluorocarbon liquids (FX-80). Anesthesiology 34:312, 1971.

AVAILABLE BLOOD COMPONENTS

COMPONENT	CONTENT	INDICATIONS	VOLUME	SHELF LIFE
Red cells a. Whole	RBC's and: WBC's, platelet debris, WBC's plasma	Red cell volume, plasma	450 ± 50 cc's	ACD 21 days CPD 28 days CPD adenine 35 days
b. Packed	Some plasma, platelet debris, WBC's	Red cell volume	200 ml RBC's	ACD 21 days CPD 28 days CPD adenine 35 days
c. Frozen	No plasma, minimal WBC's and platelet debris	Red cell volume	160-190 cc's RBC's	Frozen: ? Thawed: 24 hours
WBC concentrates	WBC's, few platelets	Agranulocytosis ? sepsis	Variable 50-100 cc's	12 hours
Platelets	Platelets, few WBC's and some plasma	Thrombocytopenia, platelet dysfunction	30-50 ml/unit	6-72 hours
Fresh frozen plasma	Plasma proteins, all coagulation factors except platelets	Bleeding from coagulation, deficiency (V, VIII), volume expansion	200-250 cc's	Thawed: 2 hours Frozen: years
Cryoprecipitate	Factors I, VIII	Hemophilia, Von Willebrand's disease, fibrinogen deficiency	25 ml	Thawed: 4-6 hours
AHG concentrate	VIII	Hemophilia	Lyophilized	Dated
Konyne, Proplex	II, VII, IX, X	Christmas disease	Lyophilized	Dated
Albumin 25%	Albumin	Volume, oncotic pressure	50 ml	3-5 years
5%	Albumin and saline	Volume, oncotic pressure	250 ml	3-5 years
Plasma protein fraction	Albumin, alpha globulin, beta globulin	Volume expansion, oncotic pressure	250 ml	3-5 years
Immune serum globulin	Gamma globulin	Disease, prophylaxis, alpha gamma globulinemia	Varies with weight	3 years
Rh_O (D) immune globulin	Gamma globulin, sensitized donors	Prevention of Rh sensitization	1-2 ml	3 years

CARDIOVASCULAR AND BIOCHEMICAL RESPONSES TO DELIBERATE HYPOTENSION

D.E. LONGNECKER

Although any of several drugs may be employeed to produce hypotension, the actions of these agents may be explained by one of two
hemodynamic mechanisms. Arterial pressure may be reduced either by
decreases in cardiac output or by decreases in peripheral vascular
resistance. While it may be uncommon for any drug to have an effect on
either the heart or the peripheral circulation exclusively, the drugs
which are used to produce hypotension act primarily by one or the other
of these mechanisms. For example, halothane produces hypotension
primarily by direct myocardial depression, while sodium nitroprusside
(SNP) and nitroglycerin (NG) act primarily on the peripheral circulation.
Among those drugs which act on the periphery, some reduce arterial
pressure primarily by dilating the arterial resistance vessels while
others have predominant effects on the venous capacitance vessels.
INFLUENCES OF DELIBERATE HYPOTENSION ON THE PERIPHERAL CIRCULATION

Both direct and indirect techniques have been used to evaluate the
actions of SNP and NG on the peripheral circulation. For the most part,
studies in laboratory animals have employed direct assessments of the
peripheral circulation, including blood flow and microvascular
diameters, while indirect techniques have been used in humans in order
to avoid the invasive nature of the direct techniques.

The peripheral circulatory effects of SNP have been determined in
the muscle microvasculature of rats. The cremasteric microvasculature
was identified according to orders of branching and the influences of
SNP were determined in both arterioles and venules before, during and
after hypotension was produced by intravenous SNP. SNP did not alter
the diameters of the larger first-order arterioles, but it dilated the

smaller fourth-order precapillary arterioles. SNP had no effect on the diameters of first-order or third-order venules. Subsequent investigations demonstrated that these veins could respond to other vasodilators, indicating that SNP acts primarily on the arteriolar bed in the muscle of rats.

The radioactive microsphere technique was used to quantitate regional blood flows during SNP-induced hypotension in rats. Cardiac output was unaltered by SNP but systemic vascular resistance was reduced by 27 percent. Cerebral blood flow declined by 23 percent and renal blood flow by 25 percent during SNP infusion, while splanchnic flow increased by 19 percent. The results suggest that SNP exerts its principal vasodilator effects primarily in the splanchnic microvasculature of rats. However, possible venous effects of this drug cannot be evaluated with the microsphere method because the mircospheres lodge in the capillaries before they reach the venous circulation. These data suggest that the brain and kidneys may be vulnerable organs for tissue ischemia during deliberate hypotension, since blood flows were significantly reduced in these organs during SNP infusion. Comparative studies for NG are unavailable, primarily because of the great difficulty in reducing blood pressure in rats with NG.

Gerson, et. al. compared the arteriolar and venous effects of SNP and NG in 20 adult patients during cardiopulmonary bypass. Each patient received three doses of SNP and three doses of NG during constant flow extracorporeal circulation. Changes in systemic arterial pressure were used as indices of the effects of the drugs on the arteriolar resistance vessels, while changes in whole body venous capacitance were estimated by observing the fluid level in the blood reservoir connected to the oxygenator circuit. The results suggested that, at least for the larger doses of SNP and NG, these drugs have differing effects on the arterioles and venules of humans. The results indicate that SNP is a more effective arteriolar dilator while NG is a more effective venous dilator. It should be emphasized that these studies were performed in humans during cardiopulmonary bypass, a highly abnormal state which produces its own alterations in circulatory control. Nevertheless, the methods used in these studies did allow a clear separation of the arterial venous circulation and the results are consistent with other observations regarding the effects of SNP and NG on the resistance and capacitance vessels.

Stinson determined the hemodynamic effects of several intravenous vasodilators in hypertensive patients immediately after open-heart operations. In patients receiving SNP, there was a 19 percent increase in cardiac index, of 33 percent reduction in systemic vascular resistance and a 26 percent reduction in pulmonary vascular resistance. In contrast, NG reduced cardiac index by 9 percent in the absence of significant changes in pulmonary vascular resistance. NG reduced arterial pressure primarily by reductions in stroke volume and cardiac index since systemic vascular resistance was not significantly altered by this drug. These results are consistent with the concept that NG acts predominantly as a venous vasodilator, resulting in a decrease in venous return and consequently a decrease in cardiac output as well. In contrast, SNP increased stroke volume and cardiac index and the reduction in arterial pressure with this drug resulted primarily from a decrease in systemic vascular resistance, indicating an arteriolar site of action for SNP. Trimethaphan, in contrast to either SNP or NG, reduced both systemic vascular resistance and cardiac index, indicating that this drug probably dilates both arterioles and venules.

Peripheral Circulatory Actions of Vasodilators in Humans with Congestive Heart Failure or Acute Myocardial Infarction.

The effects of SNP and NG on circulatory and cardiac function have been compared in patients with coronary artery disease and congestive heart failure. SNP increased both cardiac index and the ejection fraction, while NG did not alter these values. In the periphery, SNP reduced both systemic vascular resistance and forearm vascular resistance while neither of these values were altered by NG. Forearm venous tone was decreased by both SNP and NG. It was proposed that these drugs effected cardiac output primarily by their actions on the peripheral circulation. The results suggested that NG acted primarily as a venous vasodilator and that cardiac output decreased as a consequence of the venous actions of the drug. In contrast, SNP reduced arterial pressure both by decreasing systemic vascular resistance and by increasing venous capacitance, suggesting a balanced action of this drug on the arterial and venous systems.

The circulatory actions of SNP and NG have been compared in patients following acute myocardial infarction also. The drugs were not used to produce major reductions in arterial pressure, but to minimize myocardial work during the initial hours after myocardial infarction. NG produced a slightly greater reduction in pulmonary capillary wedge pressure than did SNP, but neither altered cardiac index. Systemic vascular resistance declined approximately 15 percent with either drug. The predominant effect of NG on pulmonary capillary wedge pressure was interpreted as evidence that NG affected the venous circulation, while the absence of such changes in those receiving SNP suggested that SNP did not alter the capacitance of vessels. The results were consistent with the concept that NG has a predominant venous site of action while SNP has arteriolar, or mixed arteriolar and venous, actions.

CARDIOVASCULAR AND BIOCHEMICAL RESPONSES TO DELIBERATE HYPOTENSION DURING ANESTHESIA

We studied 16 otherwise healthy patients who were undergoing operations requiring deliberate hypotension for correction of cranio-facial deformities. Anesthesia was induced with either halothane or intravenous thiopental, endotracheal intubation was accomplished, and anesthesia was maintained with halothane (0.8 % inspired) in nitrous-oxide, 60 percent. Ventilation was controlled. SNP was infused at a rate sufficient to maintain mean arterial pressure at 50-55 mmHg. We measured pH, PCO_2, PO_2, lactate, pyruvate, hematocrit and whole blood cyanide in blood samples obtained from a radial artery and from the right atrium. The duration of SNP infusion was 226±18 minutes and the total dose averaged 0.5±0.08 mg/kg. Deliberate hypotension was associated with the rapid onset of a base deficit of approximately four mEq/L and this persisted throughout. Arterial blood lactate increased (from approximately 2.5 to 4 mM/L) but this value returned to control shortly after hypotension was terminated. The changes in calculated excess lactate were similar to those for lactate alone. There were no significant changes in the PO_2 values of blood obtained from the right atrium, suggesting that cyanide toxicity did not develop in these patients. Whole blood cyanide values increased progressively throughout the period of hypotension (from an initial value of approximately 1 to a maximum value of approximately 12 µM/L) but these returned rapidly to near control values after SNP was discontinued. These results demonstrate that the metabolic effects of SNP are rapidly reversible when the infusion is terminated, at least in patients who do not receive unusually large doses of the drug. Indeed, the need for large total doses of SNP during surgery would appear to be unusual, as evidenced by the relatively low doses of SNP which were required to maintain hypotension in these patients. Both blood lactate and excess lactate values returned to normal within one hour after discontinuing SNP, although the slight base deficit persisted for at least two hours. The absence of significant increases in oxygen the tension of blood obtained from the right atrium strongly suggest that cyanide toxicity did not occur in these patients, since cyanide toxicity would be associated with decreased oxygen consumption and increased venous oxygen tension. In our patients, we were unable to demonstrate a significant correlation between the blood cyanide value and the base excess value, suggesting that acid-base changes may not be especially helpful in determining whether cyanide toxicity may be developing. We found a very good correlation between the blood cyanide concentration and dose of SNP, expressed either as the rate of infusion or as the cumulative dose of SNP administered. This suggests that recommendations to limit the infusion rate and/or total dose of SNP may be more useful to prevent cyanide toxicity than attempting to monitor indirect indicators of blood cyanide during the procedure.

SUMMARY AND CONCLUSIONS

The peripheral vascular actions of the hypotensive agents are especially difficult to interpret because the effects of the drugs themselves are often counteracted by homeostatic mechanisms which attempt to restore arterial pressure during deliberate hypotension. Thus an agent that acts primarily on the periphery to reduce arterial pressure may be counteracted by a reflex increase in heart rate and cardiac output as the body attempts to restore arterial pressure to normal values. Nevertheless, the results of a variety of studies are consistent enough to allow some generalizations. Both SNP and NG produce their hypotensive actions primarily as a result of their effects on the peripheral circulation. In animals, SNP acts primarily on the smaller precapillary arterioles and direct evidence of venous effects of this drug have not been reported. In humans, SNP exerts profound effects on systemic vascular resistance indicating a major action on the arterioles. The venous effect of SNP is not consistently evident in humans, but it is suggested by changes in ventricular filling pressures. In contrast, NG has minimal effects on the arteriolar resistance vessels but it has pronounced effects on the veins. Systemic veins are markedly dilated by SNP resulting in increased venous capacitance, decreased venous return, decreased ventricular filling pressures and, ultimately, decreased cardiac output.

With regard to the biochemical changes resulting from SNP-induced hypotension during anesthesia, the following conclusions appear to be warranted: (a) SNP-induced hypotension of at least four hours duration is well tolerated in otherwise healthy patients receiving halothane anesthesia; (b) although blood cyanide increased in all patients, this increase was relatively small and rapidly reversible when SNP was discontinued; (c) some evidence of metabolic acidosis occured during and after the SNP infusion; and (d) the best predictive indicator of blood cyanide concentration was the dose of SNP infused, not the acid-base or venous oxygen values which were obtained at regular intervals during SNP infusion. While these acid-base and oxygen tension values should be monitored carefully, it is perhaps more important to limit the total dose and rate of SNP infusion than to rely on the indirect indicators to avoid cyanide toxicity.

REFERENCES

1. Gerson JI, Allen FB, Seltzer JL, Parker FB, Markowitz AH: Arterial
    and venous dilation by nitroprusside and nitroglycerin -- is there
    a difference? Anesth Analg 61:256-260, 1982
2. Gmeiner R, Riedl J, Baumgartner H: Effect of sodium nitroprusside
    on myocardial performance and venous tone. Eur J Pharmacol
    31:287-291, 1975
3. Longnecker DE, Creasy RA, Ross DC: A microvascular site of action
    of sodium nitroprusside in striated muscle of the rat.
    Anesthesiology 50:111-117, 1979
4. Miller ED, Delaney TJ: Blood flow alteration induced by saralasin
    or sodium nitroprusside in rats. Anesthesiology 54:199-203, 1981
5. Stinson EB, Holloway EL, Derby G, Oyer PE, Hollingsworth J,
    Griepp RB, Harrison DC: Comparative hemodynamic responses to
    chloropromazine, nitroprusside, nitroglycerin, and trimethaphan
    immediately after open-heart operations. Circulation (Suppl I)
    51, 52:26-33, 1975

POSTOPERATIVE MANAGEMENT OF CARDIAC PATIENTS: CARDIAC VS. NON-CARDIAC
SURGERY

MYER H. ROSENTHAL, M.D.

The postoperative care of patients with cardiac disease regardless of
the type surgery performed exhibit certain fundamental similarities. Basic
physiologic principles must be followed and used as guidelines for the
formulation of therapeutic regimes for all organ systems. In this discussion
the subject will be divided into a systems approach covering major areas.
Attempts will be made to highlight those areas of significance to the physician caring for patients following cardiac surgery. Of note is the
author's preference and emphasis on a pathophysiologic approach supported
by appropriate monitoring with mechnical and pharmacologic treatment.

HEMODYNAMIC
The work of Otto Frank and Ernest Starling at the turn of the century
still form the basis for therapy to optimize hemodynamic function.

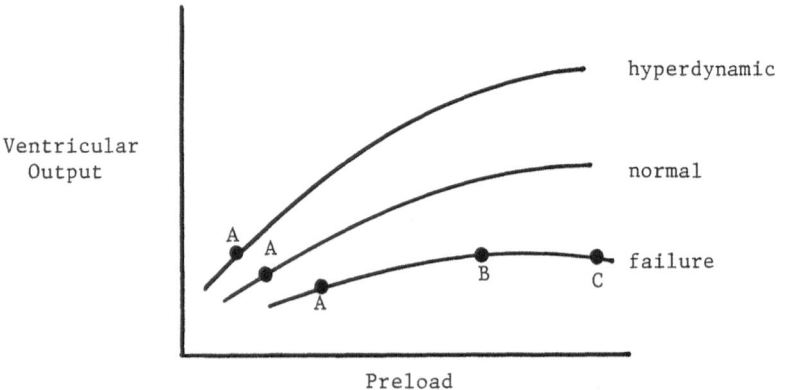

In the above diagram the Frank-Starling relationship demonstrating states of altered contractility (hyperdynamic, failure) and possible hemodynamic alterations are graphically portrayed. Points A is a hypovolemic state. Point B shows optimal preload in a failing myocardium and Point C the preload is likely excessive and the heart is failing. Based on the above a patient with low output syndrome can be examined and an estimate of etiology made.

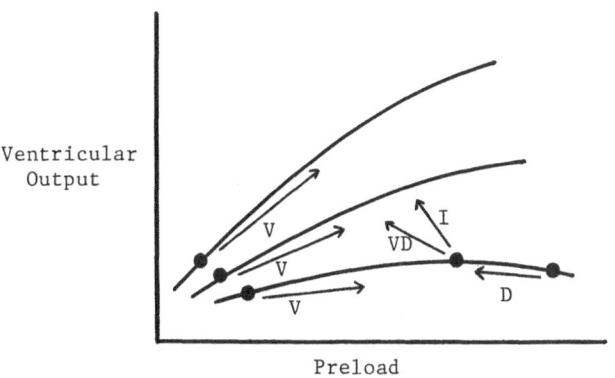

Once such a hypothesis is prepared treatment to improve cardiac output should be tried as shown above where V is volume, VD is vasodilators, I is inotropes and D is diuretics or venodilators. The response to this therapy, which should be immediately evaluated, determines the validity of the initial hypothesis, the need to continue the same regime or to modify one's therapy.

In addition to the evaluation and management of low cardiac output states, further concern, particularly in patients with coronary artery disease, is sufficient myocardial oxygenation. The relationship of myocardial oxygen consumption (preload, contractility, afterload, heart rate) to myocardial oxygen availability (coronary perfusion and arterial oxygen content) is critical. In this regard careful attention must be paid to heart rate. Tachycardia is extremely detrimental as it is responsible for marked increases in oxygen demand while decreasing diastolic time and thus oxygen supply. Careful attention therefore to all factors is necessary in avoiding oxygen supply/demand disequilibrium.

Where the above principles hold for both cardiac and non-cardiac
surgery, certain unique features pertaining to cardiac surgery deserve
further emphasis. It has been observed that following cardiopulmonary
bypass the contractile state of the heart is often depressed requiring
elevated preload and occasional inotropic support. The duration of this
decreased contractility is often between 24 and 48 hours. Early impressions
in the late 1960's led clinicians to believe that central venous (CVP) and
mean left atrial (MLAP) pressures of 20 torr were essential in the early
postoperative periods following cardiopulmonary bypass (CPB). Now, with
more critical monitoring, improved surgical and anesthetic technique as
well as means for cardiac preservation such routine practices are no longer
appropriate and individual titration of therapy based on previously described physiology is more suitable. Careful review of preoperative history
and catheterization data can be extremely beneficial in estimating postoperative requirements. Hypothermia is not uncommonly observed following
CPB resulting in high vascular resistance in the early postoperative period.
This often impedes the ability to restore intravascular volume and further
serves to reduce ventricular output.

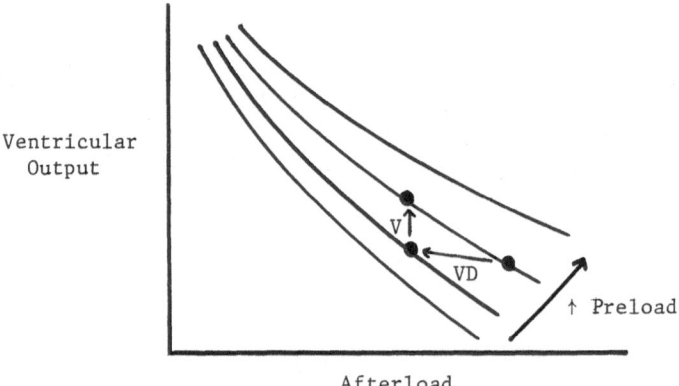

Therefore, it is fairly common to use vasodilators (VD) to decrease resistance and thus afterload accompanied by careful attention to preload with
volume (V) administration. This not only allows the physician to improve
output and perfusion but also avoids the sudden severe hypotension that
accompanies rapid rewarming.

The development of arrhythmias in the early postoperative period is also of major concern. Ventricular and atrial ectopy are often a result of potassium and hydrogen ion imbalance and careful attention to the need for potassium replacement and acid-base imbalance is essential. Trauma and edema to the conduction system may also result in varying degrees of "block" with "escape-type" rhythms requiring pacemaker assistance. One of the more common delayed complications in cardiac surgery is the appearance of supraventricular tachycardias 24 to 72 hours postoperatively. A number of pharmacologic methods have been recommended to both avoid as well as modify this factor including early digitalization, propanolol and the use of quinidine or procainamide at the first sign of atrial ectopy.

The use of mechanical assist devices to aid the weakened myocardium is increasingly apparent. Most common is the intra-aortic balloon counter-pulsation (IABP).

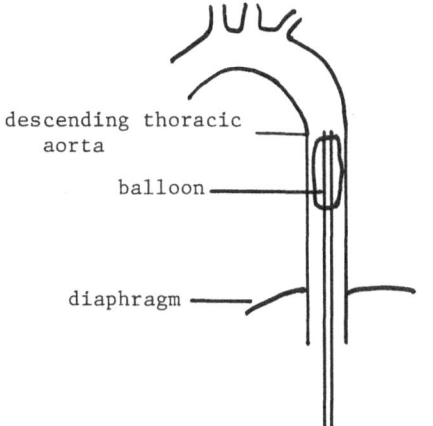

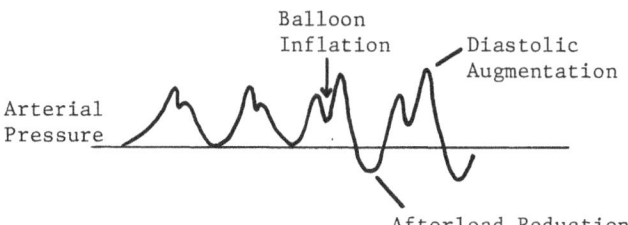

Placed in the descending thoracic aorta, most commonly via a femoral arterial cannulation, the IABP device inflates during diastole thus augmenting diastolic coronary perfusion. Critical timing is necessary for deflation to insure proper benefit of afterload reduction and non-interference with systole. Most often used to assist in weaning from CPB, the technique is also employed in cardiogenic shock and preoperatively in emergant cases of severe coronary ischemia.

One further area deserving special attention is the possible sequelae of cardiac tamponade. Continued mediastinal bleeding or sudden hemorrhage, if not adequately evacuated by drainage tubes, may lead to tamponade with sudden elevation and equalization of right and left filling pressures, fall in cardiac output and hypotension. Rapid diagnosis and immediate decompression is required.

PULMONARY

The major pathophysiologic features relevant to cardiac surgical patients are once again not dissimilar to other postoperative situations. They include abnormalities in alveolar ventilation ($\dot{V}_A$) functional residual capacity (FRC) and lung water (EVLW). The changing relationship of $\dot{V}_A$ to metabolic production of carbon dioxide during the first several hours following surgery accounts for the changes in $PaCO_2$ and pH observed. This is most often a result of rewarming and cessation of anesthesia and neuromuscular blockade. Accumulation of lung water may be based on either elevated hydrostatic pressure due to fluid overload and/or left heart failure or altered permeability. The latter takes the form of Adult Respiratory Distress Syndrome (ARDS) and has been referred to as "pump lung". This rare complication is likely due to platelet and fibrin deposition in the lung. ARDS is likely overdiagnosed in postoperative cardiac surgical patients based on normal filling pressures at the time of pulmonary artery catheterization. Placement of this monitor after EVLW has accumulated may not reflect that pathophysiology present at the initial stages. Management of this increased EVLW regardless of etiology often requires continued ventilatory support with positive-end-expired pressure (PEEP) and reduction in pulmonary capillary hydrostatic pressure (represented by pulmonary artery wedge pressure - PAW) consistant with adequate tissue perfusion. The overaggressive use of diuretics with increased EVLW can markedly reduce preload and cardiac output (C.O.) compromising renal and splanchnic perfusion. Thus the reduction in PAW must be tempered by maintenance of adequate cardiac output as shown below.

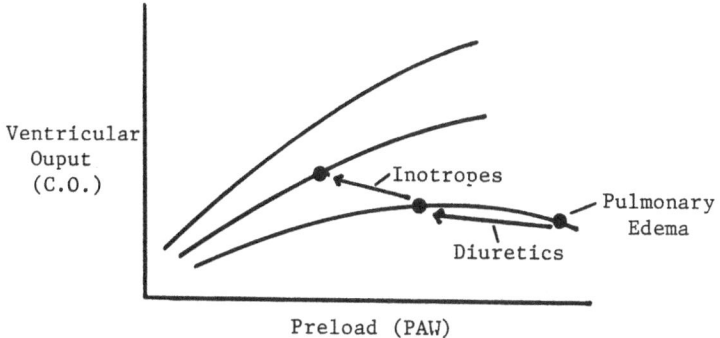

Functional residual capacity (FRC) is the most common pulmonary physiologic parameter altered by surgery and anesthesia.

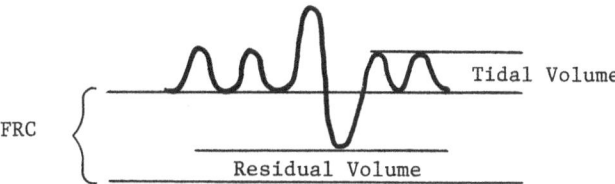

The above spirogram shows the FRC or resting volume of the lung. Most commonly depressed in the postoperative period, FRC is further effected by the collapsed position of the lungs during CPB. This depression in FRC results in a number of sequelae shown diagramatically below.

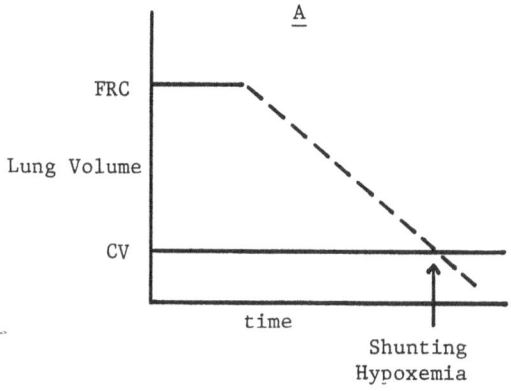

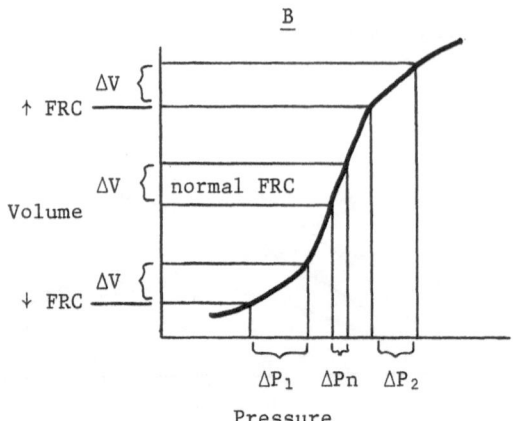

Diagram A shows the result of falling FRC as it crosses the closing volume (CV) with the development of absorption atelectasis, shunting and hypoxemia. In Diagram B the effect on compliance of changing FRC is noted. With all three ΔV's the same it should be apparent that changes in FRC either up or down result in increasing pressure change ($\Delta P_1 > \Delta Pn < \Delta P_2$) therefore compliance ($C = \Delta V/\Delta P$) decreases and respiratory work increases. The more common falls in FRC are predominantly due to atelectasis but may be aggravated by increases in EVLW. Although less common one must be alerted to the possibility of increases in FRC due to bronchospastic disease. The major treatment for low FRC is high tidal volume ventilation (12-15 cc/Kg) and the use of PEEP. Caution in applying PEEP is necessary as it may adversely effect cardiac output and is not recommended in states of elevated FRC. Improvement is based on improved compliance and oxygenation.

In evaluating pulmonary dysfunction in this specific situation of cardiac surgery, other factors including pneumothorax, hemothorax, misplaced endotracheal tubes, lobar collapse and parenchymal hemorrhage must be appreciated.

RENAL

Postoperative renal insufficiency is likely the most feared complication following major vascular and cardiac surgery. At the risk of being repetitive optimal hemodynamic management remains as the single most applicable means of avoiding this complication. As regards the cardiac surgical patient, once again several specifics need be emphasized. The intraoperative administration of mannitol will produce a marked diuresis that may result in a false reassurance of adequate function as well as a reduction in preload. The use of furosemide provides similar dilemmas. Preexisting renal dysfunction places a great deal of responsibility on the clinician to insure continued optimal perfusion and in the author's practice is a prime indication for complete hemodynamic monitoring. Hemolysis and hemoglobinuria may result from prolonged CPB and requires maintenance of high volume tubular urine flow and avoidance of acidosis which may result in crystallization and obstruction. In summary, persistant oliguria (< 0.5 cc/Kg/hr for 3+ hours) should be considered an emergency warranted aggressive diagnosis and management.

OTHER

There are a number of other areas of concern in postoperative cardiac surgical care that cannot be fully discussed in this limited text. A brief listing and comments however will follow.

Coagulation: Heparinization with questionable adequate protamine reversal, factor deficiency, platelet dysfunction, thrombocytopenia or DIC (rare) are all possible complications resulting in excessive bleeding in addition to surgical etiologies. Diagnosis and treatment is of major importance to avoid unnecessary reoperation.

Electrolytes: In addition to the previous mentioned importance of K+ and H+, attention must also be given to calcium and magnesium given their important role in myocardial contractility and arrhythmias.

Neurologic: Neurologic complications including emboli (air, etc), hypoxia-ischemia, hemorrhage and carotid occlusion may all occur. Unfortunately with the exception of evacuation of subdural or epidural hematomas, little direct intervention other then good supportive care can be offered.

Although brief this discussion has attempted to highlight those areas of specific relation to cardiac surgery. For further discussion the following suggested reading is recommended.

REFERENCES

1. Ellison N: Diagnosis and management of bleeding disorders. Anesthesiology 47:171-180, 1977.
2. Hoffman JIE, Buckberg GD: The myocardial supply:demand ratio - a critical review. Am J Card 41:327-332, 1978.

3. Kaul TK, Crow MJ, Rajah SM, et al: Heparin administration during extracorporeal circulation - heparin rebound and postoperative bleeding. J Thor CV Surg 78:95-102, 1979.
4. Kouchoukos NT, Karp RB: Management of the postoperative cardiovascular surgical patient. Am Heart J 92:513-531, 1976.
5. Lappas DG, Powell WMJ, Daggett WM: Cardiac dysfunction in the peri-operative period. Anesthesiology 47:117-137, 1977.
6. Norback CR, Tinker JH: Hypothermia after cardiopulmonary bypass in man. Anesthesiology 53:277-280, 1980.
7. Philips PA, Bregman D: Intraoperative application of intra-aortic balloon counterpulsation determined by clinical monitoring of the endocardial viability ratio. Ann Thor Surg 23:45-51, 1977.
8. Sladen RN: Management of the adult cardiac patient in the intensive care unit in Ream AK, Fogdall RP: Acute Cardiovascular Management. J.B. Lippincott CO., Philadelphia, 1982.

EARLY EXTUBATION .... FOR

MYER H. ROSENTHAL, M.D.

Before discussing those factors favoring early extubation, an examina-
tion of circumstances that have led to this "controversy" seems in order.
During the 1960's cardiac surgery established itself for the correction of
congenital anomalies as well as acquired valvular disease and septal defects.
During this period emphasis on the cardiovascular system led many physicians
to place the respiratory system "on hold" until cardiac stability was
evident. There was also concern as to the ability of the lungs to respond
to the severity of this insult. As a consequence of this reasoning, a
number of arbitrary conclusions were made and practices established. Ventilatory assist was determined to be beneficial in minimizing oxygen demands
and this coupled by a fear of a multitude of complications led to proposals
for maintaining intubation and assisted ventilation for a minimal period
of 24 hours followed by tracheostomy and continued ventilatory support if
the patient could not be weaned. Some centers advocated immediate tracheostomy at surgery due to the belief that prolonged mechanical ventilation was
an essential component for recovery. The advent of coronary artery bypass
graft surgery (CABG) brought new concerns that further continued belief in
prolonged respiratory support. The ability of the patient with severe
coronary artery disease to tolerate the stress of awakening and recovery
from anesthesia and surgery was theorized to require minimizing the strain
by maintaining heavy sedation and mechanical ventilation for up to 48 hours.
It was hoped that careful weaning after such a delay would be better tolerated without metabolic or cardiac complications and minimal increase in
oxygen demand. It should be understood that there were never any scientific
studies undertaken to verify the need for such therapy.

Over the past twenty years a number of improvements have taken place
that have caused many clinicians to question the need for the above postoperative regime. Greater understanding of physiology coupled with improved
monitoring has helped to lessen the mystique of cardiac surgery and lead

to a more realistic approach to postoperative care. The rapid reestablish-
ment of functional residual capacity using high tidal volume ventilation
and positive-end-expired pressure (PEEP) decreased the atelectasis and
shunting that required prolonged ventilatory assistance. Improved anesthesia, shorter procedures, techniques of cardiac preservation and increased
numbers of CABG patients with otherwise negative past medical history has
allowed us to tailor our postoperative care individually and provided
increasing numbers of patients who tolerate and benefit from early weaning
and extubation.

Extensive data demonstrating true benefit in comparative studies of
late versus early extubation is not available. However, a number of studies
and the author's experience demonstrate the safety and feasibility of early
extubation. It is important at this point to clarify what is meant by early
extubation. In the context of this discussion, extubation at less than
eight hours postoperatively will be considered "early". Lell and his group
demonstrated a significantly shorter duration of intensive care unit (ICU)
stay. Also, Quasha has published data showing less sedative requirement
and less cardiopulmonary morbidity following extubation at 2 ± 2 hours
postoperatively compared to 18 ± 3 hours. The experience at Stanford
Medical Center has verified the safety for early extubation, the decreased
requirement for sedation and shortened ICU stay. In addition, we have
observed a significant cost saving in overall hospital bills in patients
in whom early extubation has been possible.

Regardless of these demonstrated benefits, there is little doubt that
early extubation can be accomplished without hazard or increased morbidity
in a large portion of cardiac surgery patients. If this is accepted, it
is difficult to justify unnecessarily prolonged intubation given its own
inherent complications, including airway dislodgement, inspissation of
secretions, bacterial colonization and laryngeal trauma. In recommending
early consideration for extubation, it is assumed that careful assessment
of pulmonary as well as overall status will be accomplished. It should be
obvious that where the contention here is that subjecting all patients to
prolonged ventilatory support is inappropriate so to is the arbitrary
designation of early extubation. Individualization of care is of prime
importance in designating proper pulmonary management in the postoperative
period for any procedure.

REFERENCES

1. Cooperman LH, Mann PEG, et al: Postoperative respiratory care: A review of 65 consecutive cases of open-heart surgery on the mitral valve. J Thor CV Surg 53:504-507, 1967.
2. Klineberg PL, Geer RT, Hirsh RA, et al: Early extubation after coronary artery bypass graft surgery. CCM 5:272-274, 1977.
3. Lefemine AA, Harken DE: Postoperative care following open-heart operations: routine use of controlled ventilation. J Thor CV Surg 52:207-216, 1966.
4. Lell WA, Samuelson PN, Reves JG, et al: Duration of intubation and ICU stay after open heart surgery. S Med J 72:773-775, 1979.
5. MacRae WR, Mason AHB: Assisted ventilation in the post-bypass period. Brit J Anaesth 36:711-716, 1964.
6. Michel L, McMichan JC, Marsh HM, et al: Measurement of ventilatory reserve as an indicator for early extubation after cardiac operation. J Thor CV Surg 78:761-764, 1979.
7. Prakash O, Jonson B, Melj S, et al: Criteria for early extubation after intracardiac surgery in adults. Anesthe Analg 56:703-708, 1977.
8. Quasha AL, Loeber N, Feeley TW, et al: Postoperative respiratory care: a controlled trial of early and late extubation following coronary-artery bypass grafting. Anesthesiology 52:135-141, 1980.
9. Thung N, Herzog P, Christlieb II, et al: The cost of respiratory effort in postoperative cardiac patients. Circulation 28:552-559, 1963.
10. Zeitlin GL: Artificial respiration after cardiac surgery. Anaesthesia 20:145-155, 1965.

EARLY EXTUBATION .... AGAINST

D. DAVID GLASS, M.D.

Some have stated that there is a "controversy" regarding the
appropriate timing of extubation following cardiac surgery. It is
important to define what is meant by early extubation, and, as far as
the existence of a controversy between myself and Doctor Rosenthal,
his definition of early meaning within eight hours following cardiac
surgery eliminates any controversy that I might believe in.

I am against extubation for cardiac surgical patients (a) during
bypass, (b) prior to closure of the sternum, or (c) prior to leaving
the Operating Room!

I am also against extubation at any time that some very fundamental
principles are not followed and some elementary data is not accumulated.
Those determinants are:

I. The anesthetic technique chosen. Large doses of narcotic very
often mandate a ventilatory pattern of mechanical support simply because
of displacement of the CO_2 response curve.

II. Cardiovascular stability, particularly the absence of serious
arrhythmias, and a measured cardiac index that is less than 2 to 2.5
liters per minute. Either or both of these situations suggest that any
change in the work of breathing or any need for further resuscitative
efforts, the placement and presence of an endotrachial tube will
facilitate either. It does not mean that the patient needs to be
mechanically ventilated, which could also compromise hemodynamic function, and that CPAP or very low IMV rates may be perfectly acceptable
in these circumstances.

III. Bleeding of more than 100 ccs. per hour, certainly in the
first 6-8 hours, suggests that re-exploration is possible. The use of
positive end expiratory pressure via the endotrachial tube to potentially reduce bleeding has been controversial, but may be of some use.
Removal of the endotrachial tube before assessment of the coagulation

status seems inappropriate to me.

IV. Respiratory function. Prior to extubation of any patient, some basic guidelines should be followed which are predictive of the patient's ability to function without mechanical support. This is true, whether it be extubation following a routine postoperative intra-abdominal procedure or a patient who has been in the Intensive Care Unit for many weeks. The vital capacity should be 12-15 ccs. per kilogram. Arterial blood gases of 60% or less inspired oxygen should reflect the patient's ability to maintain a pH of 7.35 to 7.4, a CO_2 in the appropriate range, and a PO_2 of about 80.

V. There are other, perhaps peripheral, considerations which also should be looked for prior to extubation: the absence of central nervous system complications which would prevent airway maintenance; the achieving of normal body temperature which would prevent shivering and reduce oxygen consumption; or, in any patient where the intubation was technically very difficult, it is especially important that other systems are functioning appropriately.

As such, then, there is really no controversy between Doctor Rosenthal's definition and my view of management of the airway in cardiac surgical patients. When the above criteria have been met, which is frequently the case in coronary artery bypass surgery within the first 6-8 hours, it is my belief that this is perfectly appropriate to extubate these patients. But, if extubation occurs before assessment of each of the parameters can be made, then this kind of early extubation, I think, can only eventually lead to potential patient compromise.

REFERENCES

1. Cooperman LH, Mann PEG, et al: Postoperative respiratory care: A review of 65 consecutive cases of open-heart surgery on the mitral valve. J Thor CV Surg 53:504-507, 1967.
2. Klineberg PL, Geer RT, Hirsh RA, et al: Early extubation after coronary artery bypass graft surgery. CCM 5:272-274, 1977.
3. Lefemine AA, Harken DE: Postoperative care following open-heart operations: Routine use of controlled ventilation. J Thor CV Surg 52:207-216, 1966.
4. Lell WA, Samuelson PN, Reves JG, et al: Duration of intubation and ICU stay after open heart surgery. S Med J 72:773-775, 1979.
5. MadRae WR, Mason AHB: Assisted ventilation in the post-bypass period. Brit J Anaesth 36:711-716, 1964.
6. Michel L, McMichan JC, Marsh HM, et al: Measurement of ventilatory reserve as an indicator for early extubation after cardiac operation. J Thor CV Surg 78:761-764, 1979.
7. Prakash O, Jonson B, Melj S, et al: Criteria for early extubation after intracardiac surgery in adults. Anesth Analg 56:703-708, 1977.
8. Quasha AL, Loeber N, Feeley TW, et al: Postoperative respiratory care: A controlled trial of early and late extubation following coronary artery bypass grafting. Anesthesiology 52:135-141, 1980.
9. Thung N, Herzog P, Christlieb II, et al: The cost of respiratory effort in postoperative cardiac patients. Circulation 28:552-559, 1963.
10. Zeitlin GL: Artificial respiration after cardiac surgery. Anaesthesia 20:145-155, 1965.

ANESTHESIA AND CARDIAC TRANSPLANTATION

J.G. REVES, M.D.

Cardiac Transplantation History, Results, Candidates

Since 1967 cardiac transplantation has been a therapeutic approach to severe cardiac diseases. The history of clinical activity is marked by an enthusiasm and flurry of activity in the late 60's followed by a dormancy in interest and greatly reduced practice during the 70's, but there is now a resurgence in the performance of the operation. Techniques, primarily advanced at Stanford, have been developed so that the morbidity, mortality and long time survival are sufficiently good enough to justify the establishment of the procedure at institutions prepared to make the commitment of resources required to make the enterprise successful.[1-3] The encouraging 1982 Stanford survival rates for transplant that initiated the renewal activity were an overall survival of 65% at 1 year and approximately 45% at five years.[2]

Patient selection varies from institution to institution, but the guidelines used at Stanford are generally applied. These include: 1) presence of endstage cardiac disease, 2) a reasonably stable personality and social environment, 3) absence of severely elevated pulmonary vascular resistance (> 8 Wood units), 4) age under 55 years, and 5) no diabetes mellitus requiring insulin, no recent pulmonary infection or active infection.[1] It has been estimated that upon the basis of these recipient selection criteria, the number of potential heart transplant recipients in the United States probably ranges from 1000 to 5000 annually and that the limiting factor probably will be the number of cadaver donors which is estimated to be about 2000 per year.[3]

Patient Population

Most candidates for cardiac transplantation have a cardiomyopathy although some have severe ischemic heart disease, complex congenital disease or severe (often previously operated) valvular heart disease. Of the cardiomyopathies, most transplant candidates present with the dilated congestive type. Dilated congestive cardiomyopathy is the most common form of cardiomyopathy. It occurs worldwide in persons of all races, but predominates in men of middle age. It is frequently called idiopathic which suggests that the origin is not known. The fundamental pathology is that both ventricles lose their contractile properties and dilate (Fig. 1).

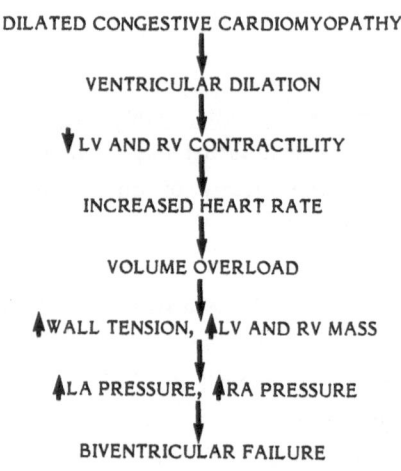

FIGURE 1. (Reproduced with permission, reference 19.)

The earliest compensatory response is an increase in ventricular volume and heart rate. Heart rate increases are more effective in augmenting the reduced cardiac output than increases in preload. Ultimately LVEDP and RVEDP rise with resultant increases in LA and RA pressure and signs of biventricular failure. The cardiac dilation that occurs increases wall tension and with further reduction of cardiac output the heart is unable to meet its increased MVO_2 requirement and fails.

During patient evaluation, it is usual to find ejection fractions in the range of 10-20%. Symptoms of left and right heart failure are present. Right heart failure usually causes anasarca and passive hepatic congestion. Notation of liver function is important including clotting abnormalities. Table I contains pertinent characteristics of our early transplant experience. Of note is the very low ejection fraction (mean 12%), elevated LVEDP (mean 26 mmHg), elevated PAP (mean 51/30) and systemic hypotension (mean 96/66). Also, most of the patients had passive hepatic congestion with deranged hepatic function tests.

Table I.

UAB CARDIAC TRANSPLANT RECIPIENTS (Nov 81-Apr 83)

| Age | Cardiac Pathology | BP | CARDIAC CATH | | | |
			PAP	LVEDP	EF	CI
12	Hypertrophic Cardiomyopathy	112/70	50/25	25	-	2.9
27	IHSS, Cardiomyopathy	90/60	47/22	18	-	-
31	Cardiomyopathy	90/70	50/40	38	10%	1.5
14	Cardiomyopathy	98/68	50/30	30	-	2.6
45	Cardiomyopathy	100/70	53/31	32	23%	1.9
18	Cardiomyopathy	100/60	50/30	32	12%	1.4
45	Cardiomyopathy	90/55	36/16	25	8%	2.3
29	Cardiomyopathy	-	-	-	7%	-
14	Complex congenital	-	-	-	-	-
28	Cardiomyopathy	95/80	65/40	34	10%	1.4
18	Cardiomyopathy	-	50/30	12	-	-
38	IHD (SP CABG)	90/60	58/35	12	-	1.3
27	(Mean)	96/66	51/30	26	12	1.9

Anesthetic Management Prior to Bypass

As with any procedure, the anesthetic management begins with the preoperative visit and patient assessment. Transplant recipients have all received some psychiatric evaluation and therapy if needed. The recipients and family are usually excitedly expectant, much like parents when labor begins, when the actual preoperative visit is made. They have waited weeks or months for the operation and the preoperative interview is facilitated by this. Little premedication is required since anxiety is not great. The patients may be NPO but we have learned that all recipients must be considered "full stomachs", and managed accordingly. After arrival at the operating room, if additional sedation with a benzodiazepine is required before induction of anesthesia, it may be given intravenously by the anesthesiologist. (Sometimes coordination of events with donor operation may postpone start of operation, particularly if the donor is at a remote hospital, and additional sedation may be required.)

The anesthetic management for patients undergoing cardiac transplantation has been reported by a number of authors.[2,4-9] Strict sterility precautions must be observed at all times because of immunosuppressive therapy. There is no consensus regarding the particular drugs used for induction and maintenance of anesthesia (Table II). The principles of patient management are: 1) rapid induction, 2) avoidance of myocardial depressant doses of anesthetic drugs, 3) maintenance of heart rate and filling pressures (the heart is

220

dependent on both to have an adequate cardiac output), and 4) possible use of vasoactive drugs which decrease afterload and/or increase contractility of the heart.

Table II.

DRUGS USED FOR INDUCTION AND MAINTENANCE OF ANESTHESIA DURING CARDIAC TRANSPLANTATION

Anesthetic Agents	Investigator (Ref #)
Thiopental/N$_2$O	Ozinsky - 1967 (4)
	Aldrete - 1969 (5)
	Paiement - 1970 (7)
Meperidine/halothane	Keats - 1969 (6)
Diazepam/morphine	Fernando - 1978 (8)
Ketamine	Reitz - 1982 (2)
Etomidate/ketamine/fentanyl	UAB

Our practice at UAB is to anesthetize patients with either ketamine (0.1 mg/kg) or etomidate (0.3 mg/kg), (Fig. 2), effect paralysis with succinylcholine (1 mg/kg) and maintain anesthesia with intermittent doses of fentanyl or ketamine as tolerated with or without N$_2$O. Pancuronium (0.1 mg/kg) is used for maintenance of paralysis. Diazepam in incremental doses of 5 mg up to 0.3 mg/kg are given as tolerated for hypnosis and amnesia prior to bypass.

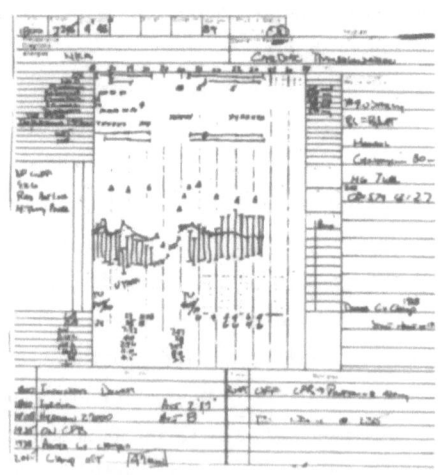

FIGURE 2.

Monitoring varies from institution to institution. These patients are as severely ill as any an anesthesiologist is likely to care for. Therefore, principles applied to the monitoring of the critically ill should apply to transplant recipients. However, infection is a constant threat to operative success and some invasive monitoring techniques (e.g. Swan-Ganz catheterizations) are not recommended apparently because of the potential for infection.[10] It is our practice to monitor EKG, radial arterial pressure, central venous pressure (CVP), and left atrial pressure (LAP), cardiac output (pulmonary artery thermister probe size 2 Fr, Wilton Webster Laboratories, placed by surgeons via the right ventricle into the PA). Therefore, we at UAB have many measures of cardiac performance, but some (LAP and CO) are not available until just prior to bypass. We have found that the hemodynamic information available is adequate for our care, though knowledge of SVR, CI, and SV might facilitate management decisions during induction and maintenance of anesthesia prior to cardiopulmonary bypass.

Post Transplant Anesthestic Management

Management after cardiac implantation is based on the same considerations as before except that there are two major differences: 1) the new heart may have had an unusual (compared with other cardiac operations) myocardial protective and ischemic course, and 2) the new heart is devoid of sympathetic and parasympathetic innervation. In our experience the donor heart has an average ischemic time of approximately two hours. Myocardial protection is with a single infusion of cold cardioplegia and the heart is transported in ice. Commonly a much longer (several minutes) than usual (about 90 seconds) time interval of rewarming is required for restoration of normal rhythm and contractility. This may be due to the long ischemic time, the residual cardioplegia, the profound cooling, or some other unknown factor. Since longer cardiac reperfusions may be expected, there is no need to begin premature pharmacologic stimulation of the recipient heart.

The denervated heart presents special problems.[11-18] Figure 3 illustrates the determinants of cardiac output and their modification by denervation. The denervated heart relies on circulating catecholamines, and appropriate preload and afterload to maintain cardiac output. Whereas the normal heart adjusts HR to augment CO, this is impossible or delayed in the denervated heart. Management of the denervated heart consists of optimizing the preload and afterload to improve CO. It is desirable to pace the heart if epicardial or endocardial wires are present. Alternatively, exogenous catecholamines may be

222

used to increase contractility and HR; apparently the acutely denervated heart is not "supra-sensitive" to catecholamines.

PHYSIOLOGY OF DENERVATED HEART

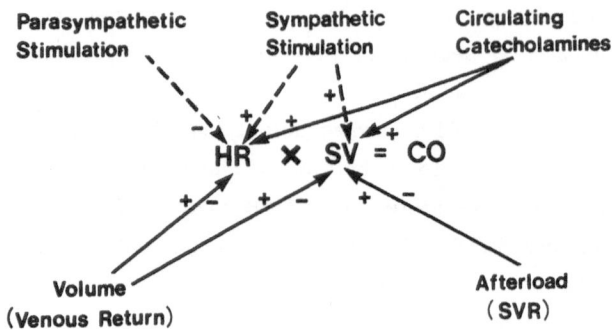

FIGURE 3. Dotted lines show loss of sympathetic and parasympathetic influence on HR and SV which are present in the normal heart. Solid lines indicate influence on normal and denervated heart. (Reproduced with permission, reference 19.)

Discontinuation of bypass usually may be accomplished with or without inotropic support. Our practice is to optimize heart rate at about 100 by pacing, achieve an LAP of about 15 mmHg, and measure the cardiac index (Fig. 4). If the cardiac index is not satisfactory (< 2.0 L/min/m^2), we begin inotropic support with isoproterenol if the SVR or PVR are elevated or with dopamine if they are normal or low. Anesthetic management is with fentanyl and N$_2$O as tolerated after bypass. Despite poor liver disease and abnormal clotting function, excessive hemorrhage is not a problem. Blood products are usually not given, though washed red cells are available should transfusion be required.

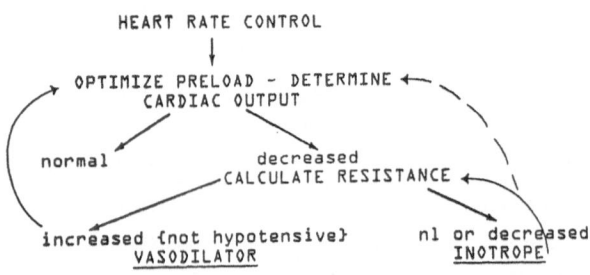

FIGURE 4.

The cardiac performance is usually good in the immediate ICU period (Fig. 5). As illustrated, only 5 of 12 patients in our early experience required inotropic support to maintain a CI over 2.0 L/min/m^2. Patients are generally extubated about 10 hours after operation and none have reported recall of operative events.

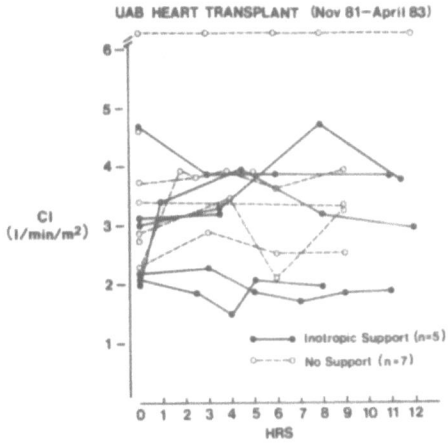

FIGURE 5.

Summary

The anesthetic management of patients requiring cardiac transplantation is a challenge to all anesthesiologists. All patients are severely ill with multiple organ system disease. The principles which apply to the management of critically ill patients are used to design the anesthetic management which takes each individual patient's requirements into account. The denervated heart requires optimal filling volume and heart rate to maximize cardiac output and inotropic support is required in the immediate post-bypass period in about 50% of cases.

References

1. Oyer PE, Stinson EB, Shumway NE: Present and future of cardiac transplantation. Ann Clin Res 13:318-326, 1981
2. Reitz BA, Fowles RE, Ream AK: Cardiac transplantation, Acute Cardiovascular Management. Edited by Ream AK, Fogdall RP. Philadelphia, J.B. Lippincott Co, 1982, pp 549-567
3. Pennock JL, Oyer PE, Beitz BA, et al: Cardiac transplantation in perspective for the future. J Thorac Cardiovasc Surg 83:168-177, 1982
4. Ozinsky J: Cardiac transplantation - the Anaesthetist's view: A case report. S Afr Med J 41:1268-1270, 1967
5. Aldrete JA, Pappas G: Anesthetic implications for simultaneous cardiorenal transplant. Anesth Analg 48:928-932, 1969
6. Keats AS, Strong MJ, Girgis KZ, Goldstein A: Observations during anesthesia for cardiac homotransplantation in ten patients. Anesthesiology 30:192-198, 1969
7. Paiement B, Wielhorski WA, Grondin P, et al: Anesthetic management in nine heart transplantations. Laval Med 41:186-190, 1970
8. Fernando NA, Keenan RL, Boyan CP: Anesthetic experience with cardiac transplantation. J Thorac Cardiovasc Surg 75:531-535, 1978
9. Garman JK: Anesthesia for cardiac transplantation. Clev Clin Q 48:142-146, 1981
10. Farman JV: Anaesthesia for transplant surgery. Int Anesthesiol Clin 16:92-119, 1978
11. Donald DE, Shepherd JT: Sustained capacity for exercise in dogs after complete cardiac denervation. Am J Cardiol 14:853-859, 1964
12. Shaver JA, Leon DF, Gray S III, Leonard JJ, Bahnson HT: Hemodynamic observations after cardiac transplantation. N Engl J Med 281:822-827, 1969
13. Campeau L, Pospisil L, Grondin P, Dyrda I, Lepage G: Cardiac catheterization findings at rest and after exercise in patients following cardiac transplantation. AM J Cardiol 25:523-528, 1970
14. Griepp RB, Stinson EB, Dong E Jr, Clark DA, Shumway NE: Hemodynamic performance of the transplanted human heart. Surgery 70:88-96, 1971
15. Stinson EB, Griepp RB, Schroeder JS, Dong E Jr, Shumway NE: Hemodynamic observations one and two years after cardiac transplantation in man. Circulation 45:1183-1194, 1972
16. Stinson EB, Caves PK, Griepp RB, Oyer PE, Rider AK, Shumway NE: Hemodynamic observations in the early period after human heart transplantation. J Thorac Cardiovasc Surg 69:264-270, 1975
17. Savin WM, Haskell WL, Schroeder JS, Stinson EB: Cardiorespiratory responses of cardiac transplant patients to graded, symptom-limited exercise. Circulation 62:55-60, 1980
18. Thomas JX Jr, Randall WC, Jones CE: Protective effect of chronic versus acute cardiac denervation on contractile force during coronary occlusion. Am Heart J 102:157-161, 1981
19. Reves JG: Anesthesia for acquired cardiac disease. 1983 Refresher Course Lectures. (in press)

THE ARTIFICIAL HEART

THEODORE H. STANLEY, M.D.

Each year almost one million people in this country die from heart disease, and more than 500,000 from coronary artery insufficiency.[1,2] The development of techniques to revascularize coronary arteries while helping many has not yet significantly decreased this mortality rate. Patients with irrepairable cardiac damage or totally sclerotic vessels cannot be helped and are doomed. One solution to this problem is the clinical application of cardiac transplantation. Unfortunately, there are not enough cardiac donors available nor are they frequently available at the right time to take care of sufficient numbers of potential recipients.[2,3] Another solution may be the development of an artificial heart.[2,3]

Although the heart is a vital organ, its function may be the simplest of all internal organs. It may, therefore, be possible for a man-made pump to take over the work of propelling blood through the vascular system. The earliest known mechanical artificial heart was made by V. P. Demikhov in Russia in 1937.[4] After unsuccessful attempts that year and later again in 1958, the project was terminated. In December, 1957, Kolff and Akutsu[5] successfully replaced the natural heart of a dog with a compressed air driven cardiac prosthesis made of polyvinyl chloride. While the animal survived only one and one-half hours, this initial work demonstrated that total cardiac replacement might some day be feasible. Since that time many other investigators throughout the world have become involved in artificial heart research. This report will attempt to briefly trace the development of artificial heart research in the last 26 years and deliniate some of the exciting results of the last 12 months.

Artificial Heart Requirements

Requirements of an artificial heart are similar to those of the natural heart and can be defined as follows:[6,7]

1. Each device must consist of two pumping systems (a right and left heart).
2. The pumping rate should be variable (60-120 strokes/minute).
3. Pump output should be variable and encompass as large a range as possible (2-20 liters/minute).
4. The range of pump outputs should be technically possible within a minimal range of input or "atrial" pressure (2-15 mm Hg).
5. Pump output should increase with increases in atrial pressure (intrinsic control).
6. The right and left pumps must be able to remain in balance, i.e. pump the same or reasonably similar volumes over a finite period of time, in spite of different input pressures and output resistances.
7. The artificial heart must be easy to insert into the chest and it obviously must be of a size so that the chest can be closed around it.
8. Different sizes of artificial hearts should exist for different sized patients.
9. The artificial heart must be made of a material which is compatible with natural tissues.
10. The pump must be made of a material and constructed in a design that does not stimulate clotting or injure red blood cells.
11. The moving parts of the pump must be able to tolerate hundreds of millions of cycles of bending, flexing or whatever other movement is essential for blood propulsion.

Pump Materials

Since a pump must move and the most physiologic movement is alternate compression and relaxation, most artificial hearts have been made of materials that can stretch or be deformed and then resume their previous form, i.e. rubbers. The most popular rubbers have been natural rubber, polyurethane, polyvinyl chloride and various silicone rubbers. While the most successful hearts up until a few years ago were made of silicone rubber, in the last two years pumps made of some of the new polyurethanes, among the strongest and non-thrombogenic of the known synthetic rubbers, have had tremendous success.[7-10]

Energy Sources

No matter what type of energy is used, it must eventually be converted into mechanical energy. Electricity is the most readily conceivable energy source to drive an artificial heart. It has been used to drive a motor,[11] an electromagnet,[12] a bellows,[13] and even piazoelectric bimorphic discs in artificial hearts.[14] Nuclear energy[15] is also a possibility for the future and has as its advantage the fact that it may be totally implantable. The most successful artificial hearts to date have been powered by compressed air delivered to the pump within the chest by tubes going through the chest wall.[16-18] One of the most exciting artifical hearts being developed for the future is the electro-hydraulic heart which in mock circulatory systems has a cardiac output capacity of more than 50 liters/min.[19,20]

Artificial Heart Driving and Control Systems

As mentioned above, artificial hearts must have a type of intrinsic control. Intrinsic artificial heart control is most easily achieved by maintaining constant or near constant mean arterial pressures. One of the most successful of these systems of intrinsic control for compressed air driven artificial hearts has been described by Kwan-Gett.[21] Basically it depends upon two direct acting 3-way solenoid valves which apply compressed air through two air drive lines during systole and exhaust air to atmosphere during diastole. The system is capable of independent frequency and percent systole control with the turn of two dials on the control module but is usually operated at a frequency of 80-110 beats per minute and a percent systole which ranges from 30-40 percent of the cardiac cycle. The control module also has independent right and left air drive line pressure controls which change the rate of rise of ventricular air pressures. With this system the rate of blood inflow and, therefore, the volume of blood entering the ventricle during each diastolic period increases with an increase in atrial pressure. This volume is expelled during the next ventricular systole. As filling of the ventricle diminishes so does stroke volume. There is thus an inherent balance between the pulmonic and systemic circulatory systems and extremes of high and low atrial and venous pressures are avoided. This is the intrinsic or automatic system of artificial heart control. In order to enhance ventricular filling volume, slightly subatmospheric (5 mm Hg) drive line pressure can also be used during diastole. The latter plus the control achieved by manually changing artificial heart rate and contractility is the extrinsic system of control that is possible with an artificial heart.[21-24]

Compressed air, which is, of course, the power of air driven artificial hearts, is brought from an air compressor to the control module. From the control module the compressed air is conveyed through the chest wall of the artificial heart recipient to the artificial ventricles by two small plastic air drive lines. This air is introduced between the rigid outer housing of the artificial heart and the softer, pliable inner blood containing chamber at pressures which are usually between 1-3 pounds per square inch (PSI) in the right ventricle and 3-6 PSI in the left. As mentioned above these pressures can be manually adjusted at any time by a turn of a dial on the control module and are a part of the extrinsic control system of the artificial heart.

Mock Circulatory Systems

Mock circulatory systems are used to test and evaluate artificial hearts before animal implantation to be sure they meet basic minimal dynamic requirements and are leak proof. Mock circulatory systems are of various designs and are of most importance when a design change occurs in an artificial heart.

Artificial Heart Designs

More than a decade ago Akutsu, upon reviewing the world's literature on the artificial heart, found that almost 40 different types of total mechanical hearts had been constructed and reported.[5] Since that time dozens of additional designs have also been evaluated. These have ranged from electromagnetic hearts, to roller type pumps with 1-3 rollers, to pendulum pumps, to bellofram pumps, to air or liquid driven sac or diaphragm hearts.[5,7,8,25-32] The most successful by far have been the sac or diaphragm air driven pumps.[7,18,19,26,27,32] The best of these have been polyurethane air driven diaphragm hearts.[17,18,25,32] These have an ovoid shape, are composed of four chambers (two atria and two ventricles), contain four Bjork-Shiley or pyrolytic carbon disc valves and weigh approximately 300 grams.

Surfaces

For a long time a most serious problem of artificial heart research involved the interaction of blood with the large foreign surface area that is part of the blood contacting surface of an artificial heart.[6] Blood clotting in the heart, around the artificial heart valves and at the junction of natural tissue and artificial materials with resultant impairment of ventricular filling and embolization of thrombi all over the organism, has been a major problem since the first hearts were implanted and until recently still was a significant problem.[6,9,10,25,30,32] Search for the ideal thrombo-resistant material is still going on. For a while it appeared that stimulation of a pseudo-intima via the use of surfaces covered with fibrils of Dacron, fetal fibroblasts, various proteins, etc., might be a solution to the problem.[16,30] However, control of intimal thickness plus breakage and embolization of pieces of the intima itself has proven to be a significant difficulty.[30,31] Recent artificial heart design changes, including the design of ventricles without seams or low flow stasis zones and further development of non-thrombogenic polyurethane smooth surfaces have greatly decreased these problems in animals (and greatly prolonged animal survival times).[16-18,25-32] Indeed, clot formation was not a problem in the first permanent artificial heart replacement in man, even after 112 days.

Artificial Heart Implantation Techniques

Fasted 85-105 kg Holstein calves serve as the experimental animals in artificial heart implantation procedures. Each is anesthetized with sodium brevital and then halothane or ketamine, has their treachea intubated and is placed in the supine or lateral positions on the operating table. Small gauge catheters are placed in a femoral artery and the internal jugular and femoral veins for operative and postoperative blood gas and pressure measurements. Large gauge cardiopulmonary bypass perfusion catheters are placed in one carotid artery and in both the superior and inferior vena cava. When cardiopulmonary bypass is started, the animals' natural hearts are removed, leaving only a small remnant of both atria. The artificial heart is sutured to these remnants of the atria and to the aorta and pulmonary artery.

As mentioned previously the artificial heart that is currently used is made of smooth polyurethane. It has an ovoid shape, is composed of four chambers and contains four artificial low profile disc or calf homograft valves. An artificial pulmonary artery made out of woven Dacron arterial graft material is attached proximally to the artificial heart above the right ventricular outflow valve and sutured distally to the natural pulmonary artery. Another piece of woven Dacron tubing connects the artificial left ventricle to the natural aorta. In some experiments the artificial pulmonary artery and left atrium of the artificial heart contain taps to which pieces of high pressure intravenous tubing are connected and brought out of the chest for mixed venous and left atrial blood sampling and pressure monitoring.

All calves are mechanically ventilated with oxygen at concentrations of 40-100 percent and volumes of 15-20 ml/kg/breath during the implantation procedure and for the first 6-24 postoperative hours. The animals are then weaned off the respirator and allowed to spontaneously breathe 30-40 percent oxygen or room air in order to maintain arterial oxygen tensions between 70-100 torr. Postoperatively, whole cow blood is given when needed to maintain hematocrits between 32-36 percent and lactated Ringer's solution in dextrose 5 percent water is used for the first 24-48 hours until the animals resume their natural diet of hay, grain and water. After 48 hours some animals are anticoagulated with coumadin, asprin and antiplatelet aggregation drugs to maintain venous clotting times approximately 2-3 times normal. However, many animals are never anticoagulated and do equally well.

Results

Success with the artificial heart has been long in coming but progress has been steady and improvements sometimes dramatic. After the first artificial heart survival of 90 minutes, it took three years (until 1960) to get an animal to survive as long as 6 hours.[11] With the air driven sac hearts of 1963, survival with an artificial heart was up to one day.[26] By 1966 survivals of two days were not uncommon.[27] However, it took until 1970 to get a 92 hour survival.[28] In 1969 the first human to receive any kind of an artificial heart survived for 64 hours until an unsuccessful cardiac transplantation was performed.[19] By early 1971 some animals were alive as long as a week after artificial heart implantation,[30] and then in April of 1972 our laboratory had a two week survivor.[31,32] In early 1974 animals began to live as long as 36 days with artificial hearts. In 1974 a calf lived three months with a total artificial heart replacing his natural heart. In 1975 calves lived longer than four months and in 1976 longer than 5 months. In 1978, and subsequently, calves have not infrequently lived more than seven months after artificial heart replacement.[17,18] All of the later animals have gained weight (as much as 200 pounds) and have been able to sustain rather severe treadmill exercise when requested to do so.

In December of 1982 a morbidly ill 100 kg dentist with idiopathic myocardiopathy in early cardiogenic shock having a cardiac output of approximately one liter/min, severe ventricular arrhythmias and a cardiac ejection fraction of 10 percent received the first permanant artificial heart placed in a human. Although his postoperative course was often stormy he survived for 112 days. During his last one and a half months of life he was able to talk, walk and exercise on a bicycle. Unfortunately, he also had severe end stage chronic pulmonary disease. This necessitated a tracheostomy for much of his post-artificial heart implantaiton existence. The latter made normal oral food intake difficult and, as a result, on his 111th postoperative day he aspirated foodstuff and later (on the 112th day) succumbed from an antibiotic induced pseudomembraneous enterocolitis.

Problems

Why has it taken so long to perfect a prosthetic heart? There have been many reasons. It took a long time to discover a good experimental animal model, one that was hardy, one for which large volumes of blood could be easily obtained and one which was readily available.[6,27] It also took a while for the right materials for making an artificial heart to become available.[9,10,25,29] Design of a device which could fit into the small space of the pericardial sac and not obstruct the great veins and still pump an output of as much as 14 liters/minute was also not easy.[30,32] Development of adequate control systems and realization that much of the success of artificial heart implantations depends on good postoperative care has only come lately.[21,32-34]

One of the biggest problems, which has previously been discussed, is that of surfaces, others have been infection[6,30] and hematologic difficulties.[33] As with any implanted prosthesis, meticulous attention to asepsis is mandatory. With the current dependence on energy sources from outside the body, meticulous aspesis is crucial. Development of self-contained power packed (electrical batteries) artificial hearts will hopefully diminish infection as a significant problem.

The Artificial Heart as a Research Model

Calves with artificial hearts are unique animal models to study the pulmonary effects of changes in cardiac dynamics. They are unique because they enable study of the pulmonary effects of non-pharmacologically induced changes of specific indices of cardiac function including cardiac rate, output and contractility. They also enable investigators to study controlled, elective changes in the ratio of right and left ventricular function. Using this model we have been able to determine that there is an ideal ratio of right and left ventricular contractility which minimizes pulmonary shunting and dead space ventilation and maximizes pulmonary compliance.[23,24,34,35] The ideal ventricular contractility ratio is associated with an ideal range of left atrial pressures and cardiac output.

The animal with an artificial heart can also be used as a model to study differential cardiovascular pharmacology, i.e. the percentage of a drug's cardiovascular effects which are due to its action on the heart as opposed to its action on the peripheral vasculature. Recent studies have demonstrated that approximately 40% of digoxin's effect on cardiac output increases in calves are due to its ability to increase venous return and decrease peripheral arterial resistance. A great deal of calcium's ability to increase cardiac output has also been shown to be due to the latter's effects on peripheral arterial resistance.[36]

The Future

What lies ahead? Although it is difficult to place this kind of research on a time table, it appears that the initial clinical studies will determine how important and what directions artificial heart research will take in the future. The first patient, although he lived only 112 days after receiving his artificial heart, was considered a significant success.

Many unexpected problems occurred including: early postoperative renal insufficiency with apparently normal cardiac outputs (6-8 liters/min); a cerebral insult of unknown etiology; a broken artificial valve; and early postoperative shivering of unknown etiology. Other problems were not entirely unexpected including: enormous early postoperative oxygen demands; problems with hemorrhage secondary to anticoagulation; and fitting problems of the artificial heart in the chest (during implantation). In spite of all these difficulties the pateint survived almost four months, had evidence of anabolic metabolism and was in good spirits for much of the time.

While there are obviously still problems with artificial heart control, energy transfer, etc., this first human inplantation was, in our opinion, an impressive success. The FDA has approved six additional artificial heart emplantation experiments in man. Perhaps by the time this manuscript is published a second or third patient will have received their artificial hearts.

REFERENCES

1. Report to the President: A National Program to Conquer Heart Disease. Cancer and Stroke 1, 1964.
2. Kolff WJ: Artificial organs and transplantation. Transplantation Proceed 9:53-63, 1977.
3. Jarvik RK: The total artificial heart. Scientific American 244: 74-80, 1981.
4. Demicohov VP: Experimental transplantation of vital organs. Translation by Basil Hugh. Consultants Bureau Enterprises, Inc., 227 West 17th Street, New York, NY, 1962.
5. Akutsu T, Kolff WJ: Permanent substitutes for valves and hearts. Trans Am Soc Artif Int Organs 4:230-234, 1958.
6. Moulopoulos SD, Jarvick R, Kolff WJ: Stange II problems in the project of the artificial heart. J Thoracic Cardiovascular Surgery 66:662-667, 1973.
7. Akutsu T: Artificial cardiac prosthesis. Cardiac Surgery. Second edition. New York, Appleton-Century-Crofts Publisher, 1972, p 671.
8. Lawson JH, Olsen DB, Hershgold E, Kolff J, Hadfield K, Kolff WJ: A comparison of polyurethane and silastic artificial hearts in 10 long survival experiments in calves. Trans Am Soc Artif Intern Organs 21:368-372, 1975.
9. Hanter SK, Gregonis DE, Colman DL, Androde JD, Kessler TR: Molecular weight characterizations of pre- and postimplant artificial heart polyurethane materials. Trans Am Soc Artif Inern Org 28: 473-477, 1982.

10. Lentz DJ, Pollock EM, Olsen DB, Andrews EJ: Prevention of intrinsic calcification in porcine and bovine xenograft materials. Trans Am Soc Artif Intern Organs 28:494-497, 1982.
11. Houston CS, Akutsu T, Kolff WJ: Pendulum type of artificial heart within the chest. Amer Heart J 59:723-730, 1960.
12. Kolff WJ, Akutsu T, Dreyer B, Norton H: Artificial heart in the chest and use of polyurethane for making hearts, valves and aortas. Trans Amer Soc Artif Int Organs 5:298-300, 1959.
13. Seidel W, Akutsu T, Mirkovitch F, Brown F, Kolff WJ: Air driven artificial hearts inside the chest. Trans Amer Soc Artif Int Organs 7:378-387, 1961.
14. Loehr ML, Kosch III WF, Singer M, et al: The piezoelectric artificial heart. Trans Amer Soc Artif Int Organs 10:147-150, 1964.
15. Norman JC, Pegg C, Sandberg G, Lee R: Effects of heat and radiation on dogs. Proc Artif Heart Prog Conf, Washington, D.C., 1969, p 901.
16. Kawai J, Peters J, Donovan F, et al: Implantation of a total artificial heart in calves under hypothermia with 10 day durvival. J Thoracic Cardiovascular Surgery 64:45-60, 1973.
17. Takaaki M, Lawson JH, Olsen DB, Fukumasu H, Daitoh N, Jarvik R, Kessler TR, Pons AB, Hastings L, Razzeca KJ, Nielsen SD, Kolff WJ: A seven-month survival of a calf with an artificial heart designed for human use. Artif Org 5:125-131, 1981.
18. Hastings WL, Aaron JL, Deneris J, Kessler TR, Pons AB, Razzeca KJ, Olsen DB, Kolff WJ: A retrospective study of nine calves surviving five months on the pneumatic total artificial heart. Trans Am Soc Artif Intern Organs 27:71-76, 1981.
19. Kolff WJ, Lawson J: Perspectives for the total artificial heart. Transplantation Proceed 11:317-324, 1979.
20. Jarvik RK: Electrical energy converters for practical human total artificial hearts - an opinion in support of electropneumatic systems. Artif Organs 7:21-24, 1983.
21. Kwan-Gett CS, Wu Y, Collan R, et al: Total replacement artificial heart and driving system with inherent regulation of cardiac output. Trans Amer Soc Artif Int Organs 15:245-250, 1969.
22. Stanley TH, Lawson J, Oster H: The pulmonary effects of changes in left ventricular contractility in calves with artificial hearts. Abstracts Amer Soc Artif Int Organs 3:69, 1974.
23. Stanley TH, Kilff WJ, Volder J, et al: The effects of isolated changes in right ventricular contractility on intrapulmonary shunting in calves with artificial hearts. Coronary Artery Medicine and Surgery, Appleton-Century Crofts, New York, 1975, Chapter 123, pp 1035-1040.
24. Stanley TH, Lunn JK, Liu WS, Gentry S: Effects of left atrial pressure on pulmonary shunt and the dead space/tidal volume ratio. Anesthesiology 49:128-135, 1978.
25. Kessler TR, Pons AB, Jarvik RK, Lawson JH, Razzeca KJ, Kolff WJ: Elimination of predilection sites for thrombus formation in the total artificial heart --- before and after. Trans Am Soc Artif Intern Organs 24:532-535, 1978.
26. Akutsu T, Mirkovitch V, Topaz SR, Kolff WJ: A sac type of artificial heart inside the chest of dogs. J Thoracic Cardiovascular Surgery 47:512-527, 1964.
27. Nose Y, Sarin CL, Klain M, et al: Elimination of some problems encountered in total replacement of the heart with an intrathoracic

mechanical pump: Venous return. Trans Amer Soc Artif Int Organs 12:301-309, 1966.

28. Takano H, Takagi H, Turner JD, et al: Problems in total artificial heart. Trans Amer Soc Artif Int Organs 17:449-455, 1971.

29. Cooley DA, Liotta D, Hallman GL, et al: First human implantation of cardiac prosthesis for staged total replacement of the heart. Trans Amer Soc Artif Int Organs 15:252-263, 1969.

30. Kwan-Gett CS, Backman DK, Donovan FM, et al: Artificial heart with hemispherical ventricles II and disseminated intravascular coagulation. Trans Amer Soc Artif Int Organs 17:474-481, 1971.

31. Stanley TH, Kilff WJ: The effects of smooth and Dacron lined silastic artificial hearts on survival, blood cell destruction, serum albumin and embolization. Surg Forum 24:171-173, 1973.

32. Jarvik R, Oster H, Olsen D, et al: Design of an elliptical ventricle and results of 26 implantations in calves. Abstracts Amer Soc Artif Int Organs 3:34, 1974.

33. Kolff J, Hershgold E, Hadfield C, Olsen DB, Lawson J, Kilff WJ: The improving hematologic picture in long-term surviving calves with total artificial hearts. Artif Organs 3:97-103, 1979.

34. Stanley TH, Liu WS, Isern-Amaral J, et al: Periodic pulmonary shunt analysis as a method of optimizing cardiac output after artificial heart implantation. Trans Amer Soc Artif Int Organs 21:353-360, 1975.

35. Stanley TH, Oster H: The pulmonary effects of changes in left ventricular contractility. Surg Forum 25:191-193, 1974.

36. Stanley TH, Isern-Amaral, et al: Peripheral vascular versus direct cardiac effects of calcium. Anesthesiology 45:46-58, 1976.